$\mathcal{B}$reastfeeding

and Diseases

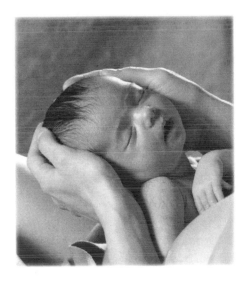

A Reference Guide

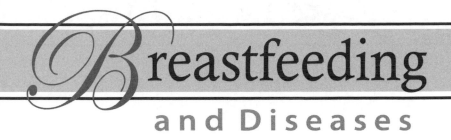

reastfeeding
and Diseases

E. Stephen Buescher, MD

Susan W. Hatcher RN, BSN, IBCLC

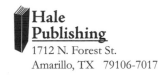

Hale
Publishing
1712 N. Forest St.
Amarillo, TX   79106-7017

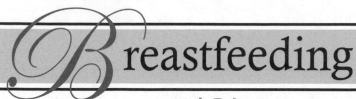

reastfeeding

and Diseases

© Copyright 2008
Hale Publishing, L.P.
1712 N. Forest St.
Amarillo, TX   79106-7017
806-376-9900 (phone)
800-378-1317 (toll-free)
806-376-9901 (Fax)
www.iBreastfeeding.com
www.hale-publishing.com

Managing Editor: Janet Rourke
Design Coordinator: Joyce Moore
Sales Director: Alicia Ingram
Production Services: Hale Publishing, L.P.

ISBN: 978-0-9815257-1-6
Library of Congress Control Number: 2008924654

Table *of* Contents

Dedication

This book is dedicated to all breastfeeding mothers and babies, and their health care providers. May every baby have the best start in life and breastfeed for as long as mother and baby desire. May every health care provider be knowledgeable about breastfeeding and do their best to preserve the breastfeeding relationship in the mothers and babies they serve.

Introduction

As healthcare providers working with breastfeeding mothers, we are continually asked whether it is safe to breastfeed in regard to various illnesses. This book was written to be a resource guide. The guide describes illnesses commonly seen in breastfeeding mothers and babies, gives suggested treatment, and discusses the disease in relation to breastfeeding. As always, when mother or baby is ill, we should try to preserve the breastfeeding relationship, unless to do so would be detrimental to the health of mother or baby. The American Academy of Pediatrics supports this position fully in their statement.

Breastfeeding and the Use of Human Milk

In 2005, the American Academy of Pediatrics published the second version of a policy statement entitled "Breastfeeding and the Use of Human Milk" (the first version was published in 1997), which outlined its organizational principles regarding breastfeeding (American Academy of Pediatrics, 2005). In this document, fifteen recommendations are made, which can be summarized as follows:

1. "Pediatricians and healthcare professionals should recommend human milk feeding for all infants in whom breastfeeding is not specifically contraindicated and should provide parents with information on the benefits and techniques of breastfeeding to ensure their feeding decision is a fully informed one."
2. "Peripartum policies and practices that optimize breastfeeding initiation and maintenance should be encouraged."
3. "Healthy infants should be placed and remain in direct skin-to-skin contact with their mothers immediately after delivery until the first feeding is accomplished."
4. "Supplements (water, glucose water, formula, and other fluids) should not be given to breastfeeding newborn infants unless ordered by a physician when a medical indication exists."
5. "Pacifier use is best avoided during the initiation of breastfeeding and should be used only after breastfeeding is well established."
6. "During the early weeks of breastfeeding, mothers should be encouraged to allow eight to twelve feedings at the breast every 24

hours, offering the breast whenever the infant shows early signs of hunger, such as increased alertness, physical activity, mouthing, or rooting."

7. "Formal evaluation of breastfeeding, including observation of position, latch, and milk transfer, should be undertaken by trained caregivers at least twice daily and fully documented in the record during each day in the hospital after birth."

8. "All breastfeeding newborn infants should be seen by a pediatrician or other knowledgeable and experienced healthcare professional at three to five days of age, as recommended by the AAP."

9. "Breastfeeding infants should have a second ambulatory visit at two to three weeks of age, so that the healthcare professional can monitor weight gain and provide additional support and encouragement to the mother during this critical period."

10. "Pediatricians and parents should be aware that exclusive breastfeeding is sufficient to support optimal growth and development for approximately the first six months of life and provides continuing protection against diarrhea and respiratory tract infection. Breastfeeding should be continued for at least the first year of life and beyond, for as long as mutually desired by both mother and child."

11. "All breastfed infants should receive 1 mg of vitamin K_1 oxide intramuscularly after the first feeding is completed and within the first six hours of life."

12. "All breastfed infants should receive 200 IU of oral vitamin D drops daily, beginning during the first two months of life and continuing until the daily consumption of vitamin D-fortified formula or milk is 500 mL."

13. "Supplementary fluoride should not be provided during the first six months of life."

14. "Mother and infant should sleep in proximity to each other to facilitate breastfeeding."

15. "Should hospitalization of the breastfeeding mother or infant be necessary, every effort should be made to maintain breastfeeding, preferably directly, or by pumping the breasts and feeding expressed milk, if necessary."

In addition to these recommendations, the AAP described the role of pediatricians and other healthcare professionals to be protecting, promoting, and supporting breastfeeding. They said pediatricians and healthcare professionals should:

- "Promote, support, and protect breastfeeding enthusiastically.
- Promote breastfeeding as a cultural norm.
- Recognize the effect of cultural diversity on breastfeeding attitudes and practices, encouraging variation that promotes and supports breastfeeding in different cultures.
- Become knowledgeable and skilled in the physiology and clinical management of breastfeeding.
- Encourage development of formal training in breastfeeding and lactation at all levels of medical training.
- Use every opportunity to provide age-appropriate breastfeeding education to children and adults.
- Work collaboratively with obstetricians to ensure women receive accurate and sufficient information throughout the perinatal period to make a fully informed feeding decision.
- Work collaboratively with the dental community to ensure that women are encouraged to continue to breastfeed and use good oral health practices.
- Promote hospital policies and procedures that promote breastfeeding.
- Provide effective breast pumps and private lactation areas for all breastfeeding mothers in ambulatory and inpatient areas of the hospital.
- Develop office practices that support and promote breastfeeding.
- Become familiar with local breastfeeding resources.
- Encourage adequate routine insurance coverage for necessary breastfeeding services and supplies.
- Develop and maintain effective communication and coordination with other healthcare professionals to ensure optimal breastfeeding education, support, and counseling.
- Advise mothers to continue their breast self-examinations on a monthly basis throughout lactation.
- Encourage the media to portray breastfeeding as positive and normative.

- Encourage employers to provide appropriate facilities and adequate time in the workplace for breastfeeding and/or milk expression.
- Encourage childcare providers to support breastfeeding and the use of expressed human milk provided by the parent.
- Support the efforts of parents and the courts to ensure continuation of breastfeeding in separation and custody proceedings.
- Provide counsel to adoptive mothers who decide to breastfeed through induced lactation.
- Encourage development and approval of government policies and legislation that are supportive to a mother's choice to breastfeed.
- Promote continued basic and clinical research in the field of breastfeeding."

Reference

American Academy of Pediatrics Section on Breastfeeding. Breastfeeding and the use of human milk. Pediatrics 115:496-506, 2005.

Acrodermatitis Enteropathica

Acrodermatitis enteropathica is a rare autosomally inherited recessive disorder of zinc transport/absorption from the digestive tract. Failure to absorb zinc from the bowel results in dermatitis, diarrhea, and alopecia, the clinical triad observed in this disorder. Onset can occur as early as two to three weeks of life, but breastfeeding usually delays the onset of the disorder until the time of weaning. On average, the age of onset in the breastfed infant is about nine months.

The disorder begins with development of rash around the mouth, nose, eyes, ears, and/or perineum. The rash is initially blister-like, then becomes dry, scaly, and crusted with sharp borders. Without treatment, the dermatitis extends to involve the cheeks, knees, elbows, buttocks, fingers, and toes (the term "acrodermatitis" means dermatitis at the edges of the body, i.e., fingers and toes), and appears eczema-like. The hair develops reddish tints, alopecia (hair loss) appears, and eye abnormalities, including conjunctivitis, blepharitis, corneal changes, and photophobia, can develop. Other accompanying findings can be chronic diarrhea, stomatitis, glossitis, growth retardation, irritability, listlessness, changes in finger and toe nails, and secondary bacterial/fungal infections. All of these changes relate to various roles of zinc in immunity and in copper, fatty acid, prostaglandin, and protein metabolism. The same constellation of clinical symptoms can be seen with inadequate zinc intake. For diagnosis, low serum zinc levels despite adequate intake plus the clinical findings described above are highly suggestive. Cases of "variant" acrodermatitis enteropathica with normal serum zinc levels have been described; these require more sophisticated methods for diagnosis than serum zinc level determinations.

A syndrome of zinc deficiency in exclusively breastfed infants has also been reported (Coelho et al., 2006; Stevens & Lubitz, 1998). The manifestations of this illness are quite similar to those of acrodermatitis enteropathica, but it either resolves when nursing ends, or it can be treated with oral zinc supplementation during breastfeeding. In some of these cases, low breastmilk zinc levels are present. Recent studies have associated maternal mutations in SLC 30A2, a gene important for zinc secretion, with some cases of transient neonatal zinc deficiency.

Treatment

Exclusive breastfeeding through the first six months of life is effective treatment for acrodermatitis enteropathica. In formula-fed infants and after weaning of breastfed infants, dietary zinc supplementation, with ongoing monitoring of serum zinc levels, can reverse most manifestations of this condition.

Breastfeeding and Acrodermatitis Enteropathica

The zinc levels in breastmilk are relatively low and cannot be increased, even if the mother increases her intake of zinc (Donellof et al., 2004). However, the bioavailability of the zinc in breastmilk is strikingly high, which likely explains the protective effect breastfeeding has on development of the clinical signs of acrodermatitis enteropathica (Lonnerdal et al., 1980). In general, the longer exclusive breastfeeding can be maintained, the less the need for zinc supplementation in this condition. Because exclusive breastfeeding provides for optimal infant growth and development through approximately six months of age, mothers of infants with acrodermatitis enteropathica should be encouraged to exclusively breastfeed their infants for the first six months of life.

Summary

Breastfeeding should be strongly encouraged for infants with acrodermatitis enteropathica.

References

Coelho S, Fernandes B, Rodriques F, Reis JP, Moreno A, Figueiredo A. Transient zinc deficiency in a breastfed, premature infant. Eur J Dermatol 16:193-195, 2006.

Domellof M, Lonnerdal B, Dewey KG, Cohen RJ, Hernell O. Iron, zinc and copper concentrations in breast milk are independent of maternal mineral status. Am J Clin Nutr 79:111-115, 2004.

Lonnerdal B, Stanislowski AFG, Hurley LS. Isolation of a low molecular weight zinc binding ligand from human milk. J Inorg Biochem 12:71-78, 1980.

Stevens J, Lubitz L. Symptomatic zinc deficiency in breast-fed term and premature infants. J Paediatr Child Health 34:97-100, 1998.

Acute Gastroenteritis

Acute gastroenteritis is a common condition with a wide variety of causes, but a narrow set of signs and symptoms: diarrhea, vomiting, and abdominal discomfort, with or without fever. Irritation, inflammation, and injury to the intestinal mucosa can produce disordered fluid absorption, carbohydrate hydrolysis, or overt fluid secretion. The large majority of episodes have infectious causes: common viral causes include rotavirus (most common), norovirus and astrovirus; common bacterial causes include *Salmonella* sp., *Shigella* sp., *Campylobacter* sp., *Escherichia coli, Yersinia enterocolitica, Clostridium difficile,* and *Vibrio* sp.; common protozoal causes include *Giardia lamblia* and *Cryptosporidium parvum*.

In the developing world, acute gastroenteritis is a major contributor to infant mortality. The younger the infant, the more readily diarrhea and vomiting can result in dehydration. If not reversed promptly, dehydration can progress to death. The agents that cause acute gastroenteritis typically are spread by the fecal-oral route. Thus, regions where sanitation is inadequate, sewage contaminates the environment, or clean water is not available are regions where acute gastroenteritis is a significant childhood problem. In these regions, breastfeeding provides both an uncontaminated source of water, and nutrients and components that are protective against many gastroenteritis pathogens. Not surprisingly, breastfeeding in these environments can enhance survival, and problems with gastroenteritis are delayed until around the time of weaning. In the developed world where environmental and water contamination are less problematic, breastfeeding still provides the advantage of components that protect against or modify the severity of acute gastroenteritis.

Treatment
In most instances, infectious gastroenteritis is a self-limiting illness that resolves over two to five days. The most crucial part of treatment for gastroenteritis is to prevent development of dehydration, which, in the absence of persistent vomiting, can usually be achieved with oral fluid intake.

Breastfeeding and Gastroenteritis
Because of the intimacy inherent to breastfeeding, transmission of agents that cause gastroenteritis from a breastfeeding mother to her infant and from

an affected infant to their mother via fecal-oral contamination are always a possibility. In the situation where a mother or infant has gastroenteritis, careful hand washing and good personal hygiene usually minimize the risk of transmission from mother-to-infant or infant-to-mother. In most instances, with the possible exception of salmonellosis, transmission of gastroenteritis agents via breastmilk (without fecal-oral contamination) from mother-to-infant is very unlikely, and therefore, breastfeeding (with good hand washing and personal hygiene) can continue.

Prevention of gastroenteritis caused by a variety of different infectious agents is one of the best documented benefits of human milk feeding (Sterling et al., 2003; Naficy et al., 1999) and one of the major reasons to continue breastfeeding after other foods are introduced into the infant's diet (American Academy of Pediatrics, 2005). Continuing to breastfeed during gastroenteritis illness in an infant is appropriate as it can provide the needed hydration and may attenuate the severity of the illness.

Summary

Breastfeeding during infant or maternal gastroenteritis can continue with appropriate attention paid to personal hygiene, good hand washing, and prevention of fecal-oral contamination.

References

American Academy of Pediatrics Section on Breastfeeding. Breastfeeding and the use of human milk. Pediatrics 115:496-506, 2005.

Naficy AB, Abu-Elyazeed R, Holmes JL, Pao MR, Savarino SJ, Kim Y, Wierzba TF, Peruski L, Lee YJ, Gentsch JR, Glass RI, Clemens JD. Epidemiology of rotavirus diarrhea in Egyptian children and implications for disease control. Am J Epidemiol 150:770-777, 1999.

Sterling LM, Richardson J, Ellis M. Clinical inquiries. Does breastfeeding protect against viral GI infections in children <2 years old? J Fam Pract 52:805-806, 2003.

Acute Otitis Media

Acute infection of the middle ear, acute otitis media, is an extremely common problem in children. Its peak incidence is in the first two years of life, and it is the most common reason for antibiotic administration in childhood. Middle ear infection usually develops following viral upper respiratory infections as a result of dysfunction of the Eustachian tube that connects the middle ear to the nasopharynx. The Eustachian tube is normally closed to prevent movement of secretions from the nasopharynx into the middle ear.

When it is closed, the middle ear develops a slightly lower pressure than is present in the pharynx. Intermittently, the Eustachian tube opens to allow both ventilation and drainage of the middle ear compartment.

This opening is the reason you hear/feel your ears "pop" when you yawn. In children, the Eustachian tube is shorter and narrower than in adults, which makes it both less effective as a barrier between the middle ear and the pharynx and more likely to become obstructed if swelling occurs in its walls. Most middle ear infections in children are preceded by an upper respiratory tract infection (usually viral), and the inflammation from this viral infection causes swelling at the nasopharyngeal exit or within the Eustachian tube. The swelling causes blockage and/or dysfunction of the tube, resulting in fluid accumulation and lowered pressure within the middle ear. If the middle ear fluid does not become superinfected by bacteria, it is called "otitis media with effusion" and will ultimately resolve when the upper respiratory infection clears and normal Eustachian tube function returns (it may require as long as three months to resolve). If the fluid becomes infected as a result of nasopharyngeal bacteria being drawn up the Eustachian tube into the middle ear, acute otitis media results.

Epidemiologic studies of the factors related to acute otitis media in the first two years of life have identified formula feeding, daycare attendance, smoking, pacifier use, male sex, and low socioeconomic status as predisposing factors for acute otitis media. Certain populations, including Native American and Inuit children, children with Trisomy 21 (Down syndrome), and those with craniofacial malformations, are more prone to developing acute otitis media. Fever and ear pain are the most common manifestations; rarely, other local or systemic infectious complications can occur.

Treatment

If left alone, approximately 75% of acute otitis media cases will resolve spontaneously over seven days. Antibiotic treatment results in a relatively small decrease in the number of clinical failures over the first seven days (about 12%), which has resulted in recent recommendations to limit early antibiotic use in the treatment of acute otitis media. In 2004, the American Academy of Pediatrics recommended that in otherwise healthy children between six months and two years of age, with non-severe illness and an uncertain diagnosis, observation without antibiotic therapy for 48-72 hours is an option (American Academy of Pediatrics, 2004).

Breastfeeding and Acute Otitis Media

Several studies have now demonstrated a protective effect of human milk feeding against acute otitis media and its associated costs (Uhari et al., 1996; Ball & Wright, 1999). The responsible mechanisms remain obscure, but could be related to fewer predisposing upper respiratory infections in the breastfed infant or to altering the invasiveness of the nasopharyngeal flora.

Summary

Breastfeeding should be continued through episodes of acute otitis media. Existing data indicate that breastfeeding provides protection against acute otitis media.

References

American Academy of Pediatrics Subcommittee on Management of Acute Otitis Media. Diagnosis and management of acute otitis media. Pediatrics 113:1451-1465, 2004.

Ball TM, Wright AL. Health care costs of formula-feeding in the first year of life. Pediatrics 103:870-876, 1999.

Uhari M, Mantysaari K, Niemela M. A meta-analytic review of the risk factors for acute otitis media. Clin Infect Dis 22:1079-1083, 1996.

Asthma

Asthma is the expression of atopic (allergic) disease in the lungs. It is an inflammatory process that results in episodic narrowing of the lower airways, the clinical hallmark of which is recurrent wheezing. The other manifestations of atopic disease are atopic dermatitis (see below) and hay fever.

Atopy is a confusing and incompletely understood biologic phenomenon involving IgE antibody, antigens, allergens, mast cells, histamine, and acute inflammation. Epidemiologic studies suggest environmental factors (temperature, tobacco smoke, pet dander) superimposed on an appropriate genetic background, along with biologic factors, such as infections, may all contribute to asthma development.

Several forms of asthma are recognized: allergic asthma, exercise-induced asthma, and occupational asthma. Allergic asthma episodes can be initiated by exposure to a variety of triggering agents: allergens, irritants, air pollution, upper and lower respiratory infections, weather changes, stress, foods, medications, or anxiety. As its name suggests, exercise-induced asthma is usually triggered by exercise. Occupational asthma is triggered by occupational exposures to allergens or irritants, and as a result, usually occurs "on the job" where the exposures occur.

In western nations, up to 10% of children less than 16 years old may be affected. In childhood asthma, 20-30% of patients develop symptoms in the first year of life, with the average age of onset being about age four. The prevalence of asthma in the US has been increasing for the past three decades, particularly in the urban, lower socioeconomic groups. In about 60% of cases, childhood asthma resolves by young adulthood.

Signs and Symptoms

While the hallmark of asthma is recurrent episodes of wheezing, recurring cough, chest tightness, and/or shortness of breath are also consistent with it. Often, a family history of asthma or other manifestations of atopy is present. Because wheezing is a prominent symptom of several common childhood respiratory infections whether or not asthma is present, making a diagnosis of "asthma" before age two is usually avoided. Beyond that age, anyone with recurrent episodes of wheezing, cough, shortness of breath, or chest tightness has a high probability of having asthma. The range of severity of asthma varies tremendously from person to person, from individuals with rare, mild asthma episodes that resolve on their own without treatment to individuals who are always symptomatic and require significant medical management to avoid the severe complications of their condition.

Treatment

Asthma treatment is based on two components: avoiding triggers and controlling symptoms. Over time, individuals or their parents recognize the triggers that cause asthma "attacks," and avoidance of these triggers is an important part of minimizing frequency of attacks. Controlling asthma symptoms usually relies on inhaled medications, which are usually divided into two groups: "controller" and "reliever/rescue" drugs. In patients requiring ongoing management of their asthma, controller drugs are taken all the time to help prevent asthma attacks. These agents predominantly target the chronic airway inflammation that is inherent in asthma. In contrast, the "reliever/rescue" drugs are taken intermittently to treat asthma attacks - they do not have a preventive role. These agents generally target the acute narrowing of the airway that occurs with an asthma attack. In some individuals with relatively mild asthma, only "reliever/rescue" medications are used when they have an occasional asthma attack. In someone with frequent asthma attacks, treatment with "controller" medications is often used to try to prevent the attacks.

Breastfeeding and Asthma Medications

For the most part, asthma medications are compatible with breastfeeding. Because asthma is an inflammatory disease, anti-inflammatory steroids (beclomethasone, flunisolide, fluticasone, triamcinolone acetinide, budesonide, prednisone, methylprednisolone), bronchodilators (albuterol, terbutaline), and mast cell stabilizers (cromolyn sodium), alone and in combinations, play crucial roles in asthma control. Most of these medications are administered by inhalation, therefore, systemic absorption and transfer of asthma treatment steroids, bronchodilator beta-adrenergic agonists, and mast cell stabilizers into the milk are low and unlikely to pose a threat to the nursing infant. If oral medications are needed to treat asthma, their ability to enter the mother's milk and potential effects on the nursing infant need to be reviewed.

Breastfeeding and Asthma

Controversy exists as to whether human milk feeding has an effect on subsequent development of asthma in a child. It is a complicated topic because of asthma definitions, certainty of asthma diagnosis, duration of follow-up for development of asthma, genetic and environmental factors, and the study methods used to examine the effects of breastfeeding. While in the past it was thought breastfeeding had a significant protective effect against development of asthma (Oddy et al., 1999), more recent information suggests that a complex relationship exists between duration of human milk feeding and development of wheezing (Fredriksson et al., 2007). Thus, if there is an effect, it is likely to be beneficial, but small (Snijders et al., 2007; Kramer et al., 2007; Matheson et al., 2007).

Summary

Asthma is a common condition in women and does not usually interfere with breastfeeding. The medications used to control and relieve asthma symptoms are usually inhaled and, therefore, are not likely to pass into the mother's milk. Oral medications for asthma need to be evaluated individually. Whether breastfeeding has effects on development of asthma in the infant is not certain. If there is an effect, it is likely to be small.

References

Fredriksson P, Jaakkola N, Jaakkola JJ. Breastfeeding and childhood asthma: a six-year population-based cohort study. BMC Pediatr 7:39, 2007.

Kramer MS, Matush L, Vanilovich I, Platt R, Bogdanovich N, et al. Effect of prolonged and exclusive breastfeeding on risk of allergy and asthma: cluster randomized trial. BMJ 335: 815, 2007.

Matheson MC, Erbas B, Balasuriya A, Jenkins MA, Wharton CL, et al. Breast-feeding and atopic disease: a cohort study from childhood to middle age. J Allergy Clin Immunol 120:1051-1057, 2007.

Oddy WH, Holt PG, Read AW, Landau LI, Stanley FJ, Kendall GE, Burton PR. Association between breast feeding and asthma in 6 year old children: findings of a prospective birth cohort study. BMJ 319:8165-819, 1999.

Snijders BE, Thijs C, Dagnelie PC, Stelma FF, Mommers M, Kummeling I, Penders J, van Ree R, van den Brandt PA. Breastfeeding duration and infant atopic manifestations, by maternal allergic status, in the first 2 years of life. J Pediatr 151: 347-351, 2007.

Atopic Dermatitis (Eczema)

Atopic dermatitis, or eczema, is the expression of atopic (allergic) disease in the skin. It is a reaction pattern of acute inflammation in the skin characterized by redness, itching, papules, vesicles, or plaques. When further irritated by itching, weeping serous discharge and crusting can develop. Atopic dermatitis can begin in infancy and is one of the most common skin disorders in childhood, estimated to affect up to 10% of children. Between 30-50% of children with atopic dermatitis will ultimately develop asthma, allergic rhinitis, or seasonal allergies (other manifestations of atopy).

Atopy is a confusing and incompletely understood biologic phenomenon involving IgE antibody, antigens, allergens, mast cells, histamine, and acute inflammation. Epidemiologic studies suggest environmental factors superimposed on an appropriate genetic background, along with biologic factors, such as infections, absence of breastfeeding, and food exposures may all contribute to its development. The clinical findings that suggest atopic dermatitis are itchy rashes that wax and wane in a setting of family history of asthma, allergic rhinitis, eczema, or food allergies.

Three forms of atopic dermatitis are commonly recognized, the manifestations of which vary by age. In infants, atopic dermatitis (infantile eczema) often presents as a papular, pruritic red rash that can progress to the point of oozing and crusting. It often begins on the cheeks, scalp, or forehead at two to six months of age. About half of the children will "outgrow" this condition by age two or three. If infantile eczema continues past two to three years of age, it usually changes to become more like atopic dermatitis that develops in older children (four to twelve years old). In this form, the rash is drier, more flaky, and tends to be accentuated on the extensor surfaces of the arms and legs and in the antecubital and popliteal fossae on the ankles and wrists. This form of eczema will improve in about 75% of cases by the teenage years. However, in 25% of cases, eczema persists into adulthood. In adults, eczema can progress to chronic changes in the skin, thickening ("elephant skin"), and lichenification, with particular involvement of the periorbital region, posterior neck, and forehead. Chronic trauma due to scratching or rubbing often leads to hyperpigmentation or to secondary bacterial superinfection.

Treatment

There are no known methods for reversing atopy. Treatment of atopic dermatitis is directed at maintaining skin hydration and minimizing itching. The former is done by application of skin moisturizing agents and avoiding strong soaps. The latter is achieved through use of antihistamines and topical corticosteroid applications. Educating the patient about the normal waxing and waning of atopic dermatitis is helpful.

Breastfeeding and Atopic Dermatitis

Women with atopic dermatitis can breastfeed. Women with a family history of atopic dermatitis should be encouraged to breastfeed because it appears to have a protective effect against allergic conditions in general, including atopic dermatitis (Kull et al., 2005).

Eczema on the nipple, areola, or breast can cause discomfort for the breastfeeding mother. Low strength topical corticosteroid ointments applied to the affected breast skin or nipple between feedings can decrease itching/pain and allow the mother to continue breastfeeding. Topical steroid treatment should be continued for no more than seven to ten days unless directed by a physician.

Summary

A mother or infant with atopic dermatitis can participate in breastfeeding. When there is a family history of atopic dermatitis, breastfeeding may decrease the severity of disease in the infant.

Reference

Kull I, Bohme M, Wahlgren CF, Nordvall L, Pershagen G, Wickman M. Breast-feeding reduces the risk for childhood eczema. J Allergy Clin Immunol 116:657-661, 2005.

Bacterial Meningitis

Meningitis is inflammation of the meninges (the membranes that surround the brain and spinal cord). The inflammation can be caused by infection (most common), by chemical irritation, or by traumatic injury. Infectious meningitis is caused by bacteria, viruses, or fungi, but bacterial meningitis is the most common and clinically significant form of this condition. Bacterial meningitis causes death in 1-5% of cases, and long term sequelae (hearing loss, seizures, cognitive deficits, or mental retardation) occur in 30-50% of survivors. Most cases occur in children less than five years old.

The causes of meningitis vary with age. In small infants, the most common causes are group B ß-hemolytic streptococci (GBS), *E. coli,* or *Listeria monocytogenes.* In hospitalized premature infants, *Klebsiella* sp, *Candida* sp., and *Staphylococcus aureus* meningitis can occur. In older infants and toddlers, *Streptococcus pneumoniae* is predominant, but *Neisseria meningitidis* and, less commonly, *Haemophilus influenzae* type B meningitis can also cause the condition. In the past, *H. influenzae* type B meningitis was quite common in infants, but the introduction of the Hib vaccine has strikingly reduced the incidence of meningitis caused by this organism.

In the summer, viral (aseptic) meningitis can become epidemic. Aseptic meningitis is usually a self-limiting condition with morbidity and mortality much lower than with bacterial meningitis. Fungal meningitis is quite uncommon unless there is underlying immunocompromise or individuals live in certain higher-risk areas.

The usual mechanism for development of meningitis is spread of the infectious agent to the meninges via the circulation. For bacterial meningitis, initial colonization of the respiratory tract is followed by entry into the circulation. The diagnosis is made by lumbar puncture (spinal tap), which allows examination and culture of the spinal fluid. Culture of the spinal fluid allows determination of the specific bacteria causing the meningitis and its antibiotic susceptibility. Diagnosis of bacterial meningitis can be difficult when antibiotics are administered before a diagnostic lumbar puncture is performed (e.g., before meningitis is suspected).

Complications of meningitis usually result from overwhelming infection, brain swelling, or blood electrolyte imbalances. The prognosis in bacterial meningitis is related to the duration of illness prior to initiation of effective therapy (the longer it was present without treatment, the worse the prognosis), the causative agent, and whether complications occur during treatment and recovery.

Bacterial meningitis is often preceded by what appears to be an upper respiratory infection, with subsequent development of central nervous system findings, or it can be part of a picture of overwhelming infection with bleeding, shock, acidosis, and respiratory failure. The clinical picture usually includes fever, irritability, lethargy, headache, vomiting, stiff neck, bulging anterior fontanelle (the soft spot on the top of an infant's head), light sensitivity, confusion, or seizures. Progression to stupor and coma can occur.

Treatment

Prompt diagnosis and treatment of meningitis are needed to optimize prognosis. Hospitalization with intensive care is often necessary, and feeding is frequently withheld until clinical stabilization is achieved. Intravenous antibiotics are the usual treatment once the diagnosis is established, usually extending for at least ten to fourteen days. For some types of bacterial meningitis, family members and close contacts are prescribed short courses of prophylactic oral antibiotics because of the possibility of spread to family members and close contacts. For prevention, vaccines against *Hemophilus influenzae* type B, *Streptococcus pneumoniae*, and *Neisseria meningitidis* are now available for use in infants, children, and adolescents.

Breastfeeding and Meningitis

Breastfeeding or provision of expressed milk while an infant has meningitis is appropriate. Several epidemiologic studies have associated breastfeeding with protection against development of bacterial meningitis caused by *H. influenzae* type B and *S. pneumoniae* (Silhverdal et al., 1999; Gessner et al., 1995).

Summary

Breastfeeding or feeding of expressed milk should continue when a child with meningitis is started on feeds. Human milk feeding protects against several types of bacterial meningitis.

References

Gessner BD, Ussery XT, Parkinson AJ, Breiman RF. Risk factors for invasive disease caused by Streptococcus pneumoniae among Alaska native children younger than two years of age. Pediatr Infect Dis J 14:123-128, 1995.

Silhverdal SA, Bodin L, Olcen P. Protective effect of breastfeeding: an ecologic study of Haemophilus influenzae meningitis and breastfeeding in a Swedish population. Int J Epidemiol 28:152-156, 1999.

Botulism, Infant

Clostridium botulinum is an anerobic microorganism that produces botulinum toxin. Botulism is the disease that results from intoxication with botulinum toxin, which usually results from consumption of the toxin in spoiled food ("food poisoning") (Sobel, 2005). A second form of botulism, "wound botulism," results from inoculation of *C. botulinum* spores into a tissue where they germinate and produce their toxin. "Infant botulism" is an intoxication with botulinum toxin, but it usually results from ingestion of *C. botulinum* spores by an infant via food or from the environment (Nevas et al., 2005), germination of the spores in the infant's intestine, production of botulinum toxin by the organisms in the infant's intestine, and absorption of the toxin from the intestine. Germination of *C. botulinum* spores in the intestine does not occur in children or adults: it is peculiar to infants and is thought to be due to differences in the intestinal environment in infants, which disappear by one year of age. In formula-fed infants, most cases occur at the time of non-formula food introductions (i.e., before six months of age), with a peak at two to four months, implying the weaning foods are the source of the spores. In breastfed infants, disease occurs somewhat later, but again, at the time of weaning.

Botulinum toxin is an extremely potent neurotoxin that blocks nerve signaling to the muscles, resulting in paralysis. "Botox" is a medical grade botulinum toxin that is used to achieve this same effect on specific muscles by local injection. One of the characteristics of the interaction of botulinum toxin with nerves is that its blocking effect can last for weeks.

C. botulinum is ubiquitous in the environment, as are its spores. Contamination of vegetables and fruits with spores is common: washing usually removes them. The most commonly recognized foods associated with development of infant botulism are honey and, prior to 1991, corn syrup.

Signs and Symptoms

The absorption of botulinum toxin from the intestine of the infant is not a sudden event; therefore, the symptoms of progressive neuromuscular blockade can vary from acute to slowly progressive, and the severity of illness can range from hard to recognize to fatal. The classic triad of findings is constipation, weakness, and poor muscle tone ("floppiness"). If symptoms progress, a symmetric, descending paralysis appears. Problems with swallowing are common because of cranial nerve involvement. An example of the clinical picture might be an infant who develops constipation and poor feeding, which progresses to poor sucking/swallowing, drooling, weak cry, poor head control, ptosis (drooping eye lids), and loss of muscular tone. Throughout, the infant remains afebrile and mentally bright which helps differentiate the picture from one of bacterial sepsis.

The diagnosis is confirmed by detection of botulinum toxin in the stool, and electromyography (tests for nerve to muscle signaling) results are characteristic.

Treatment

Treatment of infant botulism with botulinum immunoglobulin ("BabyBIG") has been shown to decrease morbidity and the duration of hospitalization for infant botulism (Long, 2001). Broad spectrum antibiotics should be avoided because lysis of intestinal Clostridia may result in abrupt release of botulinum toxin and acute worsening in neurological status (Mitchell & Tseng-Ong, 2005). The natural history of infant botulism is that it is a self-limiting illness that requires aggressive respiratory and nutritional support of the affected infant.

Breastfeeding and Infant Botulism

Recent breastfeeding and weaning are recognized epidemiologic risk factors for infant botulism (Long, 2001). This observation, so different from the usual protective role of human milk against infections, is likely due to the perturbation of the unique intestinal flora that breastfeeding supports in the infant intestine when weaning occurs. Should *C. botulinum* spores be introduced, they find this environment more conducive to their germination/growth than the stable intestinal environment of the continuously breastfed infant. Because breastfeeding babies must all eventually be weaned, this is not a situation that can be easily avoided. However, other data indicate that breastfeeding exerts a protective effect against the most severe (i.e., lethal) forms of infant botulism (Arnon et al., 1982). Thus the current recommendations of the American Academy of Pediatrics, encouragement of exclusive breastfeeding for the first six months of life (American Academy of Pediatrics, 2005) and avoidance of introduction of honey into the diet for the first year of life (AAP, 2006), can be understood.

Summary

Infants with botulism can breastfeed or receive expressed human milk. One case report describes successful breastfeeding by a mother with botulism, without transmission of botulinum toxin to her infant (Middaugh, 1978).

References

American Academy of Pediatrics, Appendix VII. Prevention of disease from potentially contamined food products. In : Pickering LK, Baker CJ, Long SS, McMillan JA (eds). Red Book: 2006 Report of the Committee on Infectious Diseases. 27th Ed. Elk Grove Village, IL: American Academy of Pediatrics; 2006: pp861-863.

American Academy of Pediatrics Section on Breastfeeding. Breastfeeding and the use of human milk. Pediatrics 115:496-506, 2005.

Arnon SS, Damus K, Thompson B, Midura DF, Chin J. Protective role of human milk against sudden infant death from infant botulism. J Pediatr 100:568-573, 1982.

Long SS. Infant botulism. Pediatr Infect Dis J 20:707-709, 2001.

Middaugh J. Botulism and breastmilk. N Engl J Med 298:343, 1978.

Mitchell WG, Tseng-Ong L. Catastrophic presentation of infant botulism may obscure or delay diagnosis. Pediatrics 116:436-438, 2005.

Nevas M, Lindstrom M, Virtanen A, Hielm S, Kuusi M, Arnon SS, Vuori E, Korkeala H. Infant botulism acquired from household dust presenting as sudden infant death syndrome. J Clin Microbiol 43:511-513, 2005.

Sobel J. Botulism. Clin Infect Dis 15:1167-1173, 2005.

Cancer

Cancer is uncontrolled growth (and sometimes spread - "metastasis") of cells originating from almost any body tissue. This growth and spread can result in damage to or death of normal tissues, replacement of functional tissue with non-functional cancer cells, or disruption or blockage of normal anatomy. Some cancers grow and spread rapidly, while others grow very slowly or remain discretely localized.

Signs and Symptoms

The signs and symptoms of cancer usually reflect the uncontrolled growth and spread (lumps, pain), damage to, or replacement of normal tissues (bleeding, fatigue, pain). Breast cancer is the type of cancer most commonly diagnosed during pregnancy and lactation, but these cases account for only 2% of all breast cancers, occurring in about 3/10,000 pregnancies. Recognition of breast cancer in this situation can be delayed because the changes in breast structure and morphology associated with pregnancy and lactation can obscure the manifestations of cancer. "Lumpy" breasts are common in lactating women. Because of this, thorough breast examination early in pregnancy should be performed to identify any pre-existing abnormalities and to establish a baseline for subsequent comparisons.

Treatment

Treatments vary with the type of cancer: surgical excision, radiation therapy, immunotherapy, hormonal therapy, or chemotherapy may be used to remove or shrink cancer cell/tumor mass and destroy cancer cells at distant locations within the body. For breast cancer, breastfeeding can continue while a suspicious mass in the breast is being evaluated, and weaning is not necessary when a breast biopsy is performed. Breastfeeding can continue on the unaffected side and on the affected side. After surgery, nursing can continue as long as the surgical site is far enough from the nipple that it is not disturbed by breastfeeding.

Breastfeeding and Cancer Therapies

The external and localized types of radiation therapy commonly used in cancer treatment are targeted at the cancer and do not affect the breastmilk. Breastfeeding can continue during these types of therapies. Internally administered radionuclide therapies (e.g., radiation emitting antibodies, ^{131}I treatment for thyroid cancer) are a contraindication to breastfeeding because the radioactivity in these treatments can potentially enter the milk and be passed to the infant. Radiation therapy directed at mammary breast cancer could affect milk production in the targeted breast due to tissue damage, but feeding can continue from the unaffected side. Chemotherapies administered as treatments for cancer may preclude breastfeeding for a short period of time while the agent "washes out." However, in consultation with the clinician, breastfeeding can likely be resumed after this period has passed. Most chemotherapy agents are administered for an immediate effect and are eliminated from the body promptly. During this "washout" period, the mother can pump and discard her milk to avoid engorgement or diminution of her milk supply. It must be emphasized that because some chemotherapy agents are more persistent and ingestion of any chemotherapy agent by the nursing infant is to be avoided, continuing to breastfeed during chemotherapy should be discussed beforehand with the physician to assure it is done in a manner safe for the infant.

Breastfeeding and Cancer

Preventative Effects in the Mother

Several studies and meta-analyses suggest that breastfeeding has a beneficial effect that decreases breast cancer in pre-menopausal women (Collaborative Group on Hormonal Factors in Breast Cancer, 2002; Bernier et al., 2000). This beneficial effect appears to be small relative to other known risk factors for breast cancer (Bernier et al., 2000).

Preventative Effects in the Infant

Several epidemiologic studies have examined breastfeeding effects on childhood cancers, and meta-analysis suggests there may be a small effect on decreasing the risks for acute lymphocytic leukemia, Hodgkin's disease, and neuroblastoma (Martin et al., 2005). However, the existing data are not strong and further well designed studies are sorely needed (Guise, 2005).

Summary

Breastfeeding may continue while a suspicious mass in the breast is being evaluated, and weaning is not necessary when a breast biopsy is performed. External and localized types of radiation therapy targeted at a breast cancer do not necessarily affect the breastmilk. Breastfeeding can continue during this type of treatment. Internally administered radiation treatments (e.g., radiation emitting antibodies, 131[1] treatment for thyroid cancer) are a contraindication to breastfeeding. Radiation therapy can affect the amounts of human milk produced by the treated breast if tissue damage from the radiation treatment occurs, but feeding can continue from the unaffected side. Chemotherapies administered as treatments for cancer usually preclude breastfeeding for a short period of time (while the agent "washes out"); however, in consultation with the clinician, breastfeeding can often be resumed after this period.

References

Bernier MO, Plu-Bureau G, Bossard N, Ayzac L, Thalabard JC. Breastfeeding and risk of breast cancer: a metaanalysis of published studies. Hum Reprod Update 6:374-386, 2000.

Collaborative Group on Hormonal Factors in Breast Cancer. Breast cancer and breastfeeding: collaborative reanalysis of individual data from 47 epidemiological studies in 30 countries, including 50302 women with breast cancer and 96973 women without the disease. Lancet 360:187-195, 2002.

Guise JM, Austin D, Morris CD. Review of case-control studies related to breastfeeding and reduced risk of childhood leukemia. Pediatrics 116: e724-e731, 2005.

Martin RM, Gunnell D, Owen CG, Smith GD. Breast-feeding and childhood cancer: a systematic review with metaanalysis. Int J Cancer 117:1020-1031, 2005.

Candidiasis

Infection caused by *Candida*, a genus of fungus, is called candidiasis or moniliasis. Infections caused by this organism usually occur on skin or mucosal surfaces (e.g., the oral, gastrointestinal, or genital mucosa). In some instances, invasive infection of deep body tissues or of the blood can occur.

In infants, the most common sites of candidiasis are the mouth and the diaper area. In breastfeeding women, the most common sites are the breasts and the genital tract. *Candida* species (*Candida* sp.) are normal inhabitants of the human gastrointestinal tract and female genitourinary tract, but their numbers are controlled by the other bacterial organisms that comprise the normal flora of those regions. If the balance between *Candida* and other intestinal flora is disrupted (as occurs with a course of antibiotic therapy or in some underlying diseases, such as diabetes), *Candida* are capable of overgrowing the remaining flora resulting in candidiasis. Normal skin is usually resistant to infection by *Candida* species, but if the skin is damaged or too moist, *Candida* can establish infection in the area of compromised skin. A rule of thumb is that *Candida* species thrive in warm, dark, and moist places. In the breastfeeding mother-infant dyad, this means candidiasis can occur in the infant's mouth ("thrush"), the infant's diaper area ("candidal diaper rash"), the mother's nipples, and possibly the deep breast tissues ("mammary candidosis"), but this is controversial. Although numerous species of Candida organisms exist, the most common human pathogens are *Candida albicans, Candida parapsilosis,* and *Candida tropicalis* - any and all of which can cause candidiasis.

Causes

Candida sp. can be isolated from the breasts of about 20-35% of lactating women, but is only rarely present (0-17%) on the non-lactating breast (Morrill et al., 2005; Zollner & Jorge, 2003). In comparison, *Candida* species are present in the mouths of about 40% of women, irrespective of their breastfeeding status, and in the mouths of 35% of breastfed infants and 67% of bottle-fed infants (2). Underlying conditions that predispose the development of candidiasis include diabetes, corticosteroid therapy, and broad-spectrum antibiotic therapy. In breastfeeding women, conditions associated with development of breast candidiasis include nipple trauma and use of plastic-lined breast pads.

Signs and Symptoms

Skin "candidiasis" infections typically appear bright red, are often pruritic (itchy) or burning, and can have "satellite lesion" (small red "bumps" set slightly away from the edges of the main red rash). Mucosal infections, such as thrush, usually appear as firmly attached whitish plaques on the mucosa that is not easily rubbed off, sometimes with associated white, cheesy-appearing discharge. Diagnosis is usually based upon appearance and associated symptoms, rather than specific culture identification of *Candida* sp., which makes the diagnosis one of presumption in many instances.

Nipple candidiasis often presents with complaints of soreness, burning, itching, and stinging pain in the nipples that persist regardless of attempts to correct positioning or latch-on techniques. The nipples may appear normal or may be pink, red, shiny, flaky, and with/without tiny pustules. More significant nipple changes, such as new cracks or previous cracking that will not heal, can also be associated with nipple candidiasis. A complaint of burning sensations or shooting pain inside the breast toward the chest wall is popularly taken to indicate "mammary candidosis," although good evidence to support this diagnostic association does not exist. Babies with oral thrush have a milky-white coating on their gums, tongue, and/or the insides of their mouths that resists removal by wiping. If the white covering can be wiped or scraped off, the underlying tissue appears red, raw, and inflamed. Babies may also have a bright red candidal diaper rash at the same time, which is due to swallowing the candida organisms in the mouth and transporting them through the GI tract to the diaper area.

Management/Treatment

Because *Candida sp.* frequently present both on the mother's breast and in the infant's mouth, treatment of one without the other is often an unsuccessful exercise. Topical antifungal treatment of surface infections using ketoconazole, nystatin, or miconazole is the first approach, with the mother applying an antifungal cream on the nipples after breastfeeding and rubbing an antifungal solution on the inside of the baby's cheeks and mouth after each feeding. Use of an antifungal cream on the infant's diaper area is also reasonable. While nystatin is a prescription medication, ketoconazole, clotrimazole, and miconazole are all available as over-the-counter preparations. These antifungal preparations are typically used for ten to fourteen days, or for at least several days after symptoms resolve. Gentian violet solution is a topical treatment option that can be used for three to five days. However, this dye causes transient staining of the tissues to which it is applied and may cause permanent staining of clothing.

If the mother does not improve over several days or suffers from recurring candidiasis, the diagnosis should be reconsidered. If still thought to be candidiasis, a prescription medication, such as oral fluconazole, may be appropriate to use. This agent is dependably active against *C. albicans*, but not as dependably active against other *Candida* sp. Ten to fourteen days of oral treatment is usually given.

During treatment, it is appropriate to try to decontaminate fomites that might harbor yeast because of contact with the infant's mouth or the mother's breasts. Items such as pacifiers, bottle nipples, teething toys can be thoroughly cleaned in hot, soapy water and boiled every day during the treatment regimen. Additionally, items such as breast pump equipment, breast shells, bra pads, or bras should be cleaned frequently as well. Breast pump attachments can be washed and boiled along with the baby items, and clothing and towels should be laundered in hot water with diluted bleach.

Candida sp. are normal inhabitants of the mouth, GI tract, and genital tract of women, so it is likely that either a mother or her infant will re-acquire

Candida sp. as normal flora after treatment. Use of good hand washing techniques, disposable bra pads, washing the infant's hands frequently if they suck their fingers/thumb, use of paper towels for hand drying, and washing infant toys regularly are all reasonable efforts to minimize re-contamination. Whether to save milk that was pumped during treatment is an open question. Freezing milk does not dependably kill *Candida* sp., so that subsequent use of milk collected during treatment should be considered as a possible means of re-introducing infection.

Breastfeeding and Candidiasis

Breastfeeding can continue during treatment for superficial breast candidiasis and during treatment of "thrush" in the infant's mouth. Efforts to prevent reinfection from contaminated equipment and/or clothing are reasonable. If treatment does not cure a condition presumed to be "candidiasis," other possible causes should be considered.

Summary

Candida sp. cause thrush in a baby's mouth, candidal diaper rash on the infant's posterior, candidiasis of the mother's nipples, and perhaps deeper infection of the breast called "mammary candidosis." *Candida* sp. are treatable with over-the-counter and prescription medications. Both mother and infant should be treated simultaneously to prevent "ping-pong" reinfection of either, and thrush can readily be re-introduced after treatment if inanimate objects in contact with either the infant's mouth or the mother's breasts or milk are not thoroughly cleaned. Mothers should continue to breastfeed during treatment for candidiasis.

References

Morrill JF, Heinig MJ, Pappagianis D, Dewey KG. Risk factors for mammary candidosis among lactating women. J Obstet Gynecol Neonatal Nurs 34:37-45, 2005.

Zollner MS, Jorge AO. *Candida* sp. occurrence in oral cavities of breastfeeding infants and in their mothers mouths and breasts. Pesqui Odontol Bras 17:151-155, 2003.

Celiac Disease

Celiac disease is a complicated autoimmune condition that affects primarily the intestines of individuals with a genetic predisposition to the condition (Chand & Mihas, 2006). It is thought to be caused by an inappropriate immune response by T-cells to a gluten protein, gliadin, which is usually eaten as part of a regular diet. IgA antibody against tissue transglutaminase develops as part of the autoimmune response and is used as a marker for the disease.

Presentation is usually in early childhood. Recent data suggest that in populations at risk for developing celiac disease autoimmunity, the timing of introduction of gluten into the diet is important: introduction in the first three months of life increased risk five fold over the risk observed when gluten was introduced between four and six months of age (Norris et al., 2005). This may partially explain the protective effect of exclusive breastfeeding in this condition.

Signs and Symptoms

The classic presenting symptom is chronic malabsorptive diarrhea, which results in failure to thrive. Other presenting manifestations can include iron deficiency anemia, osteoporosis, peripheral neuropathy, or arthritis. Other autoimmune conditions are three to ten times more common in patients with celiac disease than in the general population (Lee & Green, 2006). Biopsy of the small intestine is often the critical diagnostic test. In celiac disease, the biopsy reveals loss of intestinal villi (the major absorptive surface for the gut) plus inflammatory cell infiltration of the bowel wall.

Treatment

Removal of gluten from the diet results in amelioration of the condition and a decrease in symptoms. This usually requires removal of all wheat, barley, and rye products, resulting in a diet that is difficult to maintain. Re-introduction of even small amounts of gluten into the diet results in recurrence of the intestinal pathology and clinical symptoms.

Breastfeeding and Celiac Disease

Breastfeeding protects against development of celiac disease (Akobeng et al., 2006); the risk for children less than two years old is significantly decreased if they are still being breastfed at the time of introduction of gluten (Ivarsson et al., 2002) and is further decreased if breastfeeding continues after the introduction of gluten. The risk of developing disease also increases if gluten is introduced into the diet in large rather than moderate or small amounts.

Thus, exclusive breastfeeding through the first six months of life, with continued breastfeeding during gradual introduction of gluten into the diet is an appropriate approach to minimizing the risk of developing celiac disease in at-risk infants.

Summary

Mothers with a family history or known genetic predisposition to celiac disease should strongly consider exclusive breastfeeding for the first six months of life, with continued breastfeeding while slow introduction of gluten into the infant's diet is initiated thereafter.

References

Akobeng AK, Ramanan AV, Buchan L, Heller RF. Effect of breastfeeding on risk of coeliac disease: a systematic review and metaanalysis of observational studies. Arch Dis Child 91:39-43, 2006.

Chand N, Mihas AA. Celiac disease: current concepts in diagnosis and treatment. J Clin Gastroenterol 40:3-14, 2006.

Ivarsson A, Hernell O, Stenlund H, Persson LA. Breastfeeding protects against celiac disease. Am J Clin Nutr 75:914-921, 2002.

Lee SK, Green PH. Celiac sprue (the great modern day imposter). Curr Opin Rheumatol 18:101-107, 2006.

Norris JM, Barriga K, Hoffenberg EJ, Taki I, Miao D, Haas JE, Emery LM, Sokol RJ, Erlich HA, Eisenbarth GS, Rewers M. Risk of celiac disease autoimmunity and timing of gluten introduction in the diet of infants at increased risk of disease. JAMA 293:2343-2351, 2005.

Chlamydia

Chlamydia trachomatis is an intracellular bacteria which causes several different infectious syndromes in adults, including respiratory, genital tract, and eye infections. In infants, it is usually acquired at delivery by passage through an infected birth canal, and 25-50% of such infants develop eye infection (conjunctivitis) or pneumonia (5-20%).

Signs and Symptoms

Symptoms of genital tract infection in women can include dysuria or mucoid vaginal discharge; however, many women with genital chlamydial infections are fully asymptomatic. Chlamydial genital infection in women can cause cervicitis, salpingitis, peri-hepatitis (referred to as Fitz-Hugh-Curtis Syndrome), or pelvic inflammatory disease, with resultant infertility or ectopic pregnancy. Chlamydial genital infection in men is also often asymptomatic. Because chlamydial infection in adults is a sexually transmitted disease, treatment of both sexual partners is usually indicated.

In infants, conjunctivitis appearing shortly after birth can be caused by *Chlamydia*. Eye infection with *Chlamydia* can be accompanied by an afebrile, almost asymptomatic pneumonia caused by *Chlamydia* that appears in the first two weeks postpartum.

Diagnosis is made by either isolation of *Chlamydia* by culture or by detection of chlamydial DNA in an appropriate specimen. For men and women, urethral or endocervical swabs, respectively, are used for these purposes. In infants, swabs of eye or respiratory secretions are used. To culture *Chlamydia*, tissue culture cells must be inoculated with the clinical specimen because *Chlamydia* are obligate intracellular bacteria. Culture of urine for *Chlamydia* is also being used as a less invasive method for diagnosis in adults.

Treatment

Erythromycin or azithromycin are usually used to treat chlamydial infection. Oral treatment for genital or respiratory infections and topical (ointment) treatment for ocular infections is used. Because infection does not result in significant immunity, re-infection following successful treatment can occur.

Breastfeeding and Chlamydia

There are no data suggesting that *Chlamydia* infection can be transmitted by breastmilk. In fact, studies suggest that human colostrum is toxic to *Chlamydia* on contact (Ramsey et al., 1998; Bishai & Bishai, 1987; Skaug et al., 1982). This may explain the practice in some cultures of placing the first several drops of colostrum in the eyes of the newborn infant as a treatment for "sticky eye" (chlamydial conjunctivitis) (Bishai & Bishai, 1987). In addition, mature milk contains secretory IgA directed against *Chlamydia* (Skaug et al., 1982).

Summary

Infants with chlamydial infections may continue to breastfeed. As Chlamydia is often a sexually transmitted disease, sexual partners are usually treated simultaneously to prevent reinfection.

References

Bishai D, Bishai M. Correspondence to Editor. N Engl J Med 316:1549, 1987.

Ramsey KH, Poulsen CE, Motiu PP. The in vitro antimicrobial capacity of human colostrum against Chlamydia trachomatis. J Reprod Immunol 155-167, 1998.

Skaug K, Otnaess AB, Orstavik I, Jerve F. Chlamydial secretory IgA antibodies in human milk. Acta Pathol Microbiol Immunol Scand 90:21-25, 1982.

Chylothorax

Digestion of fat in the diet involves incorporation of the fat into structures called chylomicrons by the cells of the intestine. These chylomicrons are transported out of the gut into the lymphatic system into a fluid called chyle. Ultimately, they pass into the thoracic duct where the chyle and lymph fluid mix, from which they enter the blood stream. The thoracic duct is a delicate structure that passes from the abdomen to the upper chest where it empties into the venous system. In an adult, the thoracic duct passes up to four liters of chyle and lymph per day. If the thoracic duct is damaged or disrupted, the chyle and lymph empty into and fill the cavity into which it leaks. If disruptive in the abdomen, the resulting condition is called chylous ascites; if disruptive in the chest cavity, it is called chylothorax.

Because it compresses the lung, chylothorax is usually recognized because of respiratory distress. While "congenital" chylothorax can occur due to increased venous pressure in the infant during vaginal delivery, it more commonly results from trauma (e.g., cardiac surgery, child abuse) or occasionally from an intrathoracic process. Treatment initially involves drainage of the chylothorax to relieve respiratory distress, which hopefully allows spontaneous repair of the thoracic duct injury to stop leakage of the chyle. The negative side of chylothorax drainage is that the chyle contains a significant percentage of the calories absorbed through the intestine and many lymphocytes. Its ongoing loss through drainage results, therefore, in both a peculiar type of starvation and relative immunodeficiency.

Conservative approaches to treatment of chylothorax involve trying to minimize the amount of chyle/lymph passing through the thoracic duct to allow it to heal. This can be done through medication (octreotide) and dietary manipulation, which includes decreasing the amount of fat ingested in the diet, with its replacement by medium chain triglycerides (MCTs), which can be directly absorbed from the GI tract. Conservative treatment may require weeks to months to be effective. Surgical approaches involve obliteration of the pleural space, repair of the thoracic duct if the rupture can found, or shunting the chyle/lymph into either the circulation or the abdomen.

Breastfeeding and Chlyothorax

Fat is a prominent component in human milk, and minimizing the amount of dietary fat is an important part of conservative therapy for chylothorax. Whether breastfeeding should be curtailed as part of conservative management of chylothorax is controversial. One observational report notes successful conservative management of chylothorax can be achieved in infants with partial breastmilk feeding (Al-Tawil et al., 2000). Thus, it would seem appropriate to attempt conservative therapy while continuing to breastfeed, but if unsuccessful, switching to MCT-enriched formula may be an option before proceeding to surgical management.

Summary

Dietary adjustments are part of conservative management of chylothorax, and these include minimizing dietary fat intake. Therefore, temporary cessation of breastfeeding may be necessary. In some instances, partial breastfeeding has continued during conservative treatment, but little information on this topic is available.

Reference

Al-Tawil K, Ahmed G, Al-Hathal M, Al-Jarallah Y, Campbell N. Congenital chylothorax. Am J Perinatol 17:121-126, 2000.

Crohn's Disease (Regional Enteritis)

Crohn's disease is one of the inflammatory bowel diseases characterized by granulomatous transmural inflammation. It can involve any segment of the gastrointestinal tract (from mouth to anus) and often involves different sections of intestine with normal bowel interspersed (hence the pseudonym "regional enteritis"). This differentiates it from ulcerative colitis, which involves the rectum and colon in a continuous fashion (see Ulcerative Colitis section). In Crohn's disease, small bowel involvement is predominant (90%), in particular, the distal ileum, and misdiagnosis is common - the average time between onset of symptoms and diagnosis is one to two years.

Both genetic and environmental factors seem to be important in causing Crohn's disease. Similarities between Crohn's disease and a wasting disease in cattle, Johne's disease, which is caused by *Mycobacterium avium* subsp. *pseudotuberculosis*, have led some to propose that Crohn's disease is an infectious disease associated with this organism (Scanu et al., 2007), but this conclusion remains controversial.

Signs and Symptoms

The most common symptoms of Crohn's disease are abdominal pain, bloody diarrhea, fatigue, fever, malaise, and weight loss. Perianal disease, including fissures, abscess, or fistula development, may be associated with abdominal symptomatology. Extraintestinal inflammatory manifestations include arthritis, uveitis, aphthous stomatitis, and erythema nodosum, while anemia of chronic disease, growth failure, delayed bone maturation, and delayed sexual development can occur if the disease becomes chronic. Diagnosis is made based on clinical history, physical findings, laboratory evidence of inflammation, radiographic bowel imaging findings, and gastrointestinal endoscopy.

Treatment

Because the etiology of Crohn's disease remains obscure, treatment focuses on minimizing inflammation and reversing malnutrition. Therefore, corticosteroids, cytokine inhibitors, cytotoxic agents, and non-steroidal anti-inflammatory agents all play roles in management. Because the disease is multifocal, surgical excision of affected areas does not provide a long-term solution, but may be necessary in extreme situations.

Breastfeeding and Crohn's Disease

A recent meta-analysis of studies examining the relationship between breastfeeding and inflammatory bowel diseases (both Crohn's disease and ulcerative colitis) (Klement et al., 2004) concluded that although only a small number of high quality studies were available for analysis, development of either Crohn's disease or ulcerative colitis was less likely in individuals who were breastfed. *Mycobacterium avium* subsp *paratuberculosis* has been isolated from milk of lactating women with Crohn's disease (Naser et al., 2000). However, the significance of this observation is unknown at present, and in light of the observation that breastfeeding appears to be protective against development of Crohn's disease, a woman with Crohn's disease who wishes to breastfeed should do so with little concern.

Summary

In light of the observation that breastfeeding appears to be protective against development of Crohn's disease, a woman with Crohn's disease who wishes to breastfeed should do so with little concern.

References

Klement E, Cohen RV, Boxman J, Joseph A, Reif S. Breastfeeding and risk of inflammatory bowel disease: a systematic review with meta-analysis. Am J Clin Nutr 80:1342-1352, 2004.

Naser SA, Schwartz D, Shafran I. Isolation of Mycobacterium avium subsp paratuberculosis from breast milk of Crohn's disease patients. Am J Gastroenterol 95:1094-1095, 2000.

Scanu AM, Bull TJ, Cannas S, Sanderson JD, Sechi LA, Dettori G, Zanetti S, Hermon-Taylor J. Mycobacterium avium subspecies paratuberculosis infection in irritable bowel syndrome and comparison with Crohn's disease and Johne's diseases: common neural and immune pathogenicities. J Clin Microbiol 45:3883-3890, 2007.

Cystic Fibrosis

Cystic fibrosis (CF) is an inherited abnormality of chloride transport that leads to chronic lung and pancreatic disease in most cases. It is inherited in an autosomal recessive pattern and affects approximately 1/2500 births in Whites and approximately 1/17,000 births in Blacks.

Originally called "mucoviscidosis of the pancreas," this descriptive name clearly identifies the major problem in CF: production of extremely thick (viscous) and sticky secretions by multiple body organs (especially the lung, pancreas, and bowel) that are difficult to clear. The inability to pass these secretions results in obstruction of the passages, most frequently the airways, pancreatic tract, and biliary tract, resulting in injury to the lungs, pancreas, and liver. The clinical expression of CF is highly variable. Individuals who remain essentially asymptomatic throughout most of their lives have been reported, as have infants who develop severe morbidities in the first days of life. The life expectancy in CF depends largely on the severity of its manifestations.

Signs and Symptoms

While the ways in which CF can present in older children are highly variable, the typical neonatal presentation is meconium ileus - which occurs in about 15% of infants with CF. In this condition, the infant is unable to pass meconium because it is very thick and sticky, resulting in bowel obstruction. If the child with CF is not recognized during the newborn period, the typical young child presentation of CF is one of poor weight gain, passage of bulky, foul-smelling stools, and repeated lower respiratory infections associated with coughing and wheezing. Continuous hunger may be noted by some mothers (because the children do not absorb the calories they consume), or some note a salty taste to the skin (a result of the high sodium chloride (table salt) content in the sweat of patients with CF). Approximately two-thirds of patients with CF are diagnosed by their first birthday, but up to 10% may go undiagnosed until adolescence or adulthood.

The diagnosis is usually established by performing a sweat test. Strikingly elevated levels of sodium chloride in sweat is a hallmark of CF. The downside of this test is that collection of adequate amounts of sweat from small infants may be problematic. Alternatively, genetic tests are available for identification of some CF variants, which is useful when a known variant of CF is present in a family. In general, the earlier the diagnosis is established, the better the outlook for the child because end-organ damage in the lungs or pancreas is less.

CF is often a relentless disease with progressively more morbidity occurring as the patient passes through childhood, adolescence, and adulthood. Progressive lung disease due to chronic pneumonia caused by *Staphylococcus aureus* and *Pseudomonas aeruginosa* and progressive pancreatic insufficiency leading to chronic malnutrition and diabetes mellitus are common. In the "mucoviscidosis of the pancreas" era, death in infancy or early childhood was the rule. As the 21st century opens, median survival is into the third decade of life, largely due to institution of therapies for recurrent pneumonia and aggressive steps to prevent malnutrition.

Treatment

No cure for CF is known. Therapeutic regimes include antibiotic therapy for pulmonary infections, mucolytics, and pancreatic enzyme replacement. Organ transplantation is used in some instances of end-stage disease. Gene therapy remains an interesting, but largely elusive goal.

Breastfeeding and Cystic Fibrosis

Women with CF can breastfeed, but attention must be paid to their personal health and nutritional status. There is no broad consensus as to its risks/benefits in regard to the mother with CF. Across the U.S., 11% of cystic fibrosis centers recommend breastfeeding, 8% recommend against it, 42% recommend it on the basis of the health status of the mother, and 32% leave it to the preference of the mother (Luder et al., 1990). Colostrum and breastmilk from mothers with CF have normal concentrations of sodium (Shiffman et al., 1989). Concentrations of milk protein, fat, and sugars are normal in mothers with mild pulmonary disease (Michel & Mueller, 1994). Mothers with mild pulmonary disease can maintain their own weight while breastfeeding, and their milk can support growth in healthy infants (Michel & Mueller, 1994).

Breastfeeding the Infant with CF

Breastfeeding appears to provide the same benefits to the infant with CF as it supplies to infants without this condition. Therefore, breastfeeding of the infant with CF is to be encouraged. However, caloric intake adequate to support appropriate growth may not be achieved because of the caloric waste that occurs in CF, and supplementation with pancreatic enzyme preparations and/or hydrolyzed formula may be appropriate.

Summary

In an infant with CF, breastfeeding is encouraged. The mother with mild CF produces milk with normal concentrations of sodium, milk protein, fat, and sugars. Mothers with mild CF should maintain their weight and be assured that their milk can support growth of normal infants.

References

Luder E, Kattan M, Tanzer-Torres G, Bonforte RJ. Current recommendations for breastfeeding in cystic fibrosis centers. Am J Dis Child 144:11534-1156, 1990.

Michel SH, Mueller DH. Impact of lactation on women with cystic fibrosis and their infants: a review of five cases. J Am Diet Assoc 94:159-165, 1994.

Shiffman ML, Seale TW, Flux M, Rennert OR, Swender PT. Breast-milk composition in women with cystic fibrosis: report of two cases and a review of the literature. Am J Clin Nutr 49:612-617, 1989.

Diabetes Mellitus

Diabetes mellitus is a chronic condition that results from complete or relative deficiency of insulin, producing ineffective carbohydrate and lipid metabolism. It is classified into two types: type 1 (10%) in which insulin replacement is required, and type 2 (90%) in which either insulin secretion is present but inadequate or the tissues are resistant to the action of insulin. Insulin is produced by the beta cells of the pancreas in response to elevations in blood sugar (glucose). Production and circulation of insulin has the effect of moving glucose out of the blood into cells where it is used as fuel for cellular function. In type 1 diabetes, there is physical destruction/loss of pancreatic beta cells, which results in requirement for exogenous insulin to control glucose metabolism. Type 1 diabetes is the form usually diagnosed in childhood or adolescence and appears to have a genetic component. It is the form that is associated with development of serious chronic complications, such as peripheral vascular disease, renal disease, neuropathy, or autoimmune disorders. Type 2 diabetes is often associated with obesity and, until recently, usually presented in adulthood. In type 2 diabetes, either insulin is present but its production is diminished, or it is present but the responsiveness of cells to its actions (i.e., transporting glucose into the cell) is diminished.

Gestational diabetes is predominantly the type 2 form, producing impairment of glucose tolerance in approximately 2% of pregnancies in previously healthy women. Gestational diabetes usually presents during the second or third trimester when hormones antagonistic to the actions of insulin Ask author to name a couple reach peak levels. While gestational diabetes usually disappears at the time of birth, its development identifies women at risk for type 2 diabetes because 30-40% of previously healthy women who develop gestational diabetes go on to develop type 2 diabetes within ten years. Although gestational diabetes is frequently a mild disease, an aggressive approach to treatment is usually taken to prevent potentially serious complications of macrosomia and postpartum hypoglycemia in the fetus/infant.

Signs and Symptoms

The classic signs of type 1 diabetes mellitus are weight loss, polyphagia, polyuria, polydipsia, and lethargy, all related to hyperglycemia. The clinical picture of continued/increased urination in someone who appears ill and who has poor oral intake, as well as dehydration, is a typical presentation of this form of diabetes. The diagnosis is established by demonstration of hyperglycemia in the face of urinary ketones.

In type 2 diabetes, obesity is common and the diagnosis is most frequently made by demonstration of abnormally high blood glucose responses to an oral glucose challenge (called a glucose tolerance test).

Treatment

Treatment of type 1 diabetes is by administration of insulin to maintain normal blood glucose levels. This usually includes careful monitoring of blood glucose levels, as well as dietary management and exercise. In type 2 diabetes, oral medications may be used to increase insulin secretion when it is inadequate or to overcome resistance to its effects at the cellular level. Weight loss and exercise also figure prominently in management. Medications, such as chlorpropamide, tolbutamide, glypizide, and glyburide, are commonly used to enhance insulin production, while metformin and pioglitazone are used to overcome insulin resistance.

Breastfeeding and Diabetes Medications

Administration of exogenous insulin to lactating mothers with type 1 diabetes is not a problem as far as transfer into milk is concerned because the insulin molecule does not effectively enter the milk. Because breastmilk production comes at the expense of the mother's nutrients and calories, plasma glucose levels in lactating women with type 1 diabetes are on average lower than those in women who do not have diabetes, resulting in a reduced need for insulin in some type 1 diabetic mothers who breastfeed.

The use of oral hypoglycemic medications or insulin resistance modifying medications by breastfeeding mothers with type 2 diabetes is incompletely studied and not well understood. The American Academy of Pediatrics approves the use of tolbutamide in breastfeeding women, but many of the newer agents have not been studied. Current recommendations say other hypoglycemic medications are probably safe, but due to lack of information, close observation of both mother and infant are recommended. One report has examined the bioavailability of metformin, an insulin resistance modifying agent, in human milk and concluded that only a small percentage (about 0.3%) of the maternal dose passed into milk (Briggs et al., 2005). The authors proposed that this dose should not be significant for the nursing infant; however, they acknowledge that no clinical data are available.

Breastfeeding and Diabetes

Glucose and insulin homeostasis are better controlled in normal women who are lactating. Based on epidemiologic studies, a relationship exists between the duration of lactation and the risk of subsequent development of type 2 diabetes in the mother. Recent data from two large studies indicate that for each additional year of lactation, the risk decreases by 15% on average (Stuebe et al., 2005). A recent review of breastfeeding, type 2 diabetes, and gestational diabetes summarizes the existing data on this subject (Taylor et al., 2005).

Diabetic women can breastfeed (Ferris et al., 1988). Their establishment of lactation is slightly slower (Hartmann & Cregan, 2001), and they appear to have higher caloric intake needs to maintain their lactation, lower fasting blood glucose, and more of a predisposition toward mastitis (Ferris et al., 1988). The milk produced by women with insulin-dependent diabetes has slightly elevated levels of glucose and sodium, but other components are not different from non-diabetic women (Butte et al., 1987).

Infants of diabetic mothers are more often delivered by cesarean section (Webster et al., 1995) because of macrosomia (large size), and they have a tendency toward hypoglycemia that often requires intravenous fluids to maintain their blood glucose levels immediately postpartum. Despite this, diabetic mothers can be successful at breastfeeding (Webster et al., 1995). In epidemiologic studies, one study suggests that breastmilk consumption during the first week by infants of diabetic mothers increases their risk of becoming overweight in later childhood, implying a "window" for nutritional programming may exist in these infants (Buinauskiene et al., 2004). In the longer term, weak positive correlations are reported for duration of breastfeeding and glucose control in two-to five-year-old children of diabetic mothers (Webster et al., 1995). When children who develop type 1 diabetes are compared to controls, those with a history of prolonged breastfeeding (at least twelve months) had about half the risk seen in children who were breastfed for one to three months. Children who were not breastfed had about twice the risk relative as those breastfed for one to three months (Malcova et al., 2005).

Summary

Lactation has an epidemiologic association with prevention of type 2 diabetes later in life. Mothers with diabetes mellitus are capable of breastfeeding, and lactation in diabetic mothers is associated with lower fasting glucose levels. The milk produced by diabetic mothers has mildly increased levels of glucose and sodium, but is fully capable of supporting their infants. In epidemiologic studies, the risk that children of diabetic mothers will develop abnormal glucose tolerance is slightly decreased by breastfeeding. For children in general, prolonged breastfeeding is associated with lower risk, and no breastfeeding is associated with higher risk of developing type 1 diabetes. Mothers with diabetes should be strongly encouraged to breastfeed because human milk likely provides some protection against development of diabetes in their children.

References

Briggs GG, Ambrose PJ, Nageotte MP, Padilla G, Wan S. Excretion of metformin into breast milk and the effect on nursing infants. Obstet Gynecol 105:1437-1441, 2005.

Buinauskiene J, Baliutaviciene D, Zalinkevivius R. Glucose tolerance of 2- to 5-yr-old offspring of diabetic mothers. Pediatr Diabetes 5:143-146, 2004.

Butte NF, Garza C, Burr P, Goldman AS, Kennedy K, Kitzmiller JL. Milk composition of insulin-dependent diabetic women. J Pediatr Gastroenterol Nutr 6:936-941, 1987.

Ferris AM, Dalidowitz CK, Ingardia CM, Reece EA, Fumia FD, Jensen RG, Allen LH. Lactation outcome in insulin-dependent diabetic women. J Am Diet Assoc 88:317-322, 1988.

Hartmann P, Cregan M. Lactogenesis and the effects of insulin-dependent diabetes mellitus and prematurity. J Nutr 131:3016S-3020S, 2001.

Malcova H, Sumnik Z, Drevinek P, Venhacova J, Lebl J, Cinek O. Absence of breastfeeding is associated with the risk of type 1 diabetes: a case control study in a population with rapidly increasing incidence. Eur J Pediatr 7:1-6, 2005.

Rodekamp E, Harder T, Kohlhoff R, Franke K, Dudenhausen JW, Plagemann A. Long-term impact of breastfeeding on body weight and glucose tolerance in children of diabetic mothers: role of the late neonatal period and early infancy. Diabetes Care 28:1457-1462, 2005.

Stuebe AM, Rich-Edwards JW, Willett WC, Manson JE, Michels KB. Duration of lactation and the incidence of type 2 diabetes. JAMA 294:2601-2610, 2005.

Taylor JS, Kacmar JE, Nothnagle M. Lawrence RA. A systematic review of the literature associating breastfeeding with type 2 diabetes and gestational diabetes. J Am Col Nutr 24:320-326, 2005.

Webster J, Moore K, McMullan A. Breastfeeding outcomes for women with insulin dependent diabetes. J Hum Lact 11:195-200, 1995.

Galactosemia

Galactosemia is an autosomal recessive disorder in which metabolism of galactose is deranged due to absence of a specific enzyme, galactose-1-phosphate uridyl transferase. The absence of this enzyme prevents conversion of galactose to glucose, resulting in elevated levels of galactose and galactose by-products, which can be toxic. The primary sugar in both breastmilk and cow's milk-based infant formula, lactose, is a disaccharide composed of glucose and galactose. Hence, for the infant with galactosemia, feeding of either breastmilk or cow's milk derived infant formula results in toxic effects from galactose accumulation.

Signs and Symptoms

The classical presentation of galactosemia in an infant receiving lactose in their diet mimics sepsis, with findings of jaundice, hypoglycemia, hepatosplenomegaly, vomiting, bleeding, lethargy, and failure to thrive. For unknown reasons, infants with galactosemia also have a predilection for development of true sepsis caused by *Escherichia coli*. If not recognized, progressive liver disease, cirrhosis, liver failure, and mental retardation may develop. Death can result from untreated galactosemia.

Treatment

Early recognition and treatment by instituting a lactose/galactose-free diet is lifesaving. Testing for galactosemia is now part of the routine newborn screening done in the neonatal period - these tests have a turn-around time of one to two weeks. If galactosemia is suspected clinically, testing the infant's urine for "reducing sugars" (using a Clinitest strip or similar test) will reveal their presence, which raises the suspicion for galactosemia. Specific testing for galactose in the urine is definitive. To avoid development of neuro-cognitive deficits, the disease must be recognized in the first ten days of life and a diet without lactose/galactose instituted, such as soy-based infant formula.

Breastfeeding and Galactosemia

Breastfeeding an infant with galactosemia is absolutely contraindicated. The galactosemic infant must receive a diet without lactose or galactose in it. Breastfeeding by a mother with galactosemia is infrequent because hypogonadism with ovarian failure is common in adult females with the condition (Kaufman et al., 1981). However, pregnancy and successful delivery can occur, and breastmilk from such mothers contains adequate amounts of lactose (Forbes et al., 1988; Brivet et al., 1989). However, probably depending upon whether the galactose metabolic defect is complete or partial in the mother, the lactosemia/lactosuria that normally develops in late pregnancy/lactation may result in elevated blood levels of toxic lactose metabolites. In one reported case, lactation was successful (Forbes et al., 1988), while in another, lactation had to be stopped with bromocriptine in the first week because of increasing blood levels of toxic by-products (Brivet et al., 1989).

Summary

Breastfeeding an infant with galactosemia is absolutely contraindicated. There has been one reported case of successful lactation by a mother with galactosemia.

References

Brivet M, Raymond JP, Konopka P, Odievre M, Lemonnier A. Effect of lactation in a mother with galactosemia. J Pediatr 115:280-282, 1989.

Forbes GB, Barton LD, Nicholas DL, Cook DA. Composition of milk produced by a mother with galactosemia. J Pediatr 113:90-91, 1988.

Kaufman FR, Kogut MD, Donnell GN, Goebelsmann U, March C, Koch R. Hypergonadotrophic hypogonadism in female patients with galactosemia. N Engl J Med 304:994-998, 1981.

Gonorrhea

Neisseria gonorrhea is a Gram negative, diplococcal bacterium that causes a sexually transmitted disease called gonorrhea that usually is manifested by the purulent drainage from either the cervix or the urethra. Disseminated forms of disease can develop in the face of genital tract infection, and birth through an infected genital tract can result in neonatal infection involving the eyes (ophthalmia neonatorum), oral mucous membranes, or can cause sepsis and disseminated infection. Applying silver nitrate or erythromycin ointment in the eyes of the newborn infant after birth is done to prevent gonococcal eye infection.

Signs and Symptoms

In adults, purulent drainage from the genital tract is highly suggestive of gonorrhea. The urethral or vaginal/cervical discharge is typically thick and shows polymorphonuclear leukocytes with intracellular Gram negative diplococci - this picture provides a presumptive diagnosis. Associated complaints include dysuria (pain on urination) in both sexes and abnormal menses in females. Longer term complications in females are pelvic inflammatory disease or salpingitis that can lead to infertility or ectopic pregnancy. Disseminated disease is typically associated with skin lesions and polyarticular arthritis. Development of right upper quadrant pain may indicate development of gonococcal peri-hepatitis, also referred to as Fitzhugh-Curtis syndrome. If gonococcal genital infection is suspected, the throat should be cultured for the organism as well as the genital tract.

In infants, thick purulent conjunctivitis appearing two to four days after birth is typical of ophthalmia neonatorum, and the Gram stain of the eye secretions shows polymorphonuclear leukocytes and intracellular organisms. Other forms of neonatal infection, such as meningitis, sepsis, endocarditis, or arthritis, are also described, as are infections at the sites of scalp electrode placement of fetal scalp blood sampling.

Diagnosis is usually made by culture using Thayer-Martin agar (a culture material that will suppress the growth of other genital tract flora). Alternatively, some institutions utilize DNA probe technologies to detect *N. gonorrhea* nucleic acid in genital tract samples or in urine samples.

Treatment

Penicillin G had been the treatment of choice for gonorrhea until approximately 15 years ago, but the spread of penicillinase-producing strains has resulted in the use of single doses of ceftriaxone as the treatment of choice for uncomplicated gonorrhea. Because genital tract chlamydial infection accompanies gonorrhea in approximately 50% of cases, it is recommended that treatment for gonorrhea be accompanied by simultaneous treatment for *Chlamydia*.

Breastfeeding and Gonorrhea Medications

Although several options for treatment of uncomplicated gonorrhea are listed in the current CDC guidelines for treatment of sexually transmitted diseases (CDC, 2007), typically uncomplicated gonorrhea in an adult is treated with a single intramuscular dose (125 mg) of ceftriaxone - which is also approved for use in breastfeeding mothers by the American Academy of Pediatrics. Several options for concomitant treatment for chlamydial infection are also listed (CDC, 2007), but typically, 1 gram of azithromycin by mouth is the most common treatment used. Treatment of gonococcal infection in the newborn utilizes parenterally administered cefotaxime or ceftriaxone, the duration of which depends on the severity and extent of infection.

Breastfeeding and Gonorrhea

Treatment of gonorrhea should be initiated as soon as it is recognized. If a breastfeeding woman is diagnosed with gonorrhea, there is risk of transmission to the infant only because of the intimacy of the breastfeeding process. Reports of infection due to contact with secretions or drainage from infected mucosal surfaces exist. Therefore, an infected mother should be cautioned to pay close attention to her personal hygiene to prevent transmission to her infant. *Neisseria gonorrhea* has never been demonstrated to be passed in breastmilk.

Summary

Neisseria gonorrhea infection in a mother can be passed to her infant at the time of birth or through infant contact with infected mucosal surfaces.

Reference

CDC. Update to CDC's Sexually Transmitted Diseases Treatment Guidelines, 2006: Fluoroquinolones no longer recommended for treatment of gonococcal infections. MMWR (April 13, 2007) 56(14);332-336. http://www.cdc.gov/mmwr/preview/mmwrhtml/mm5614a3.htm?s_cid=mm5614a3_e.

Group A Streptococcal Pharyngitis (Strep Throat)

Streptococcus pyogenes (Group A ß-hemolytic streptococcus) is a Gram positive coccus with a predilection for the upper respiratory tract, explaining why it is commonly spread by oral secretions or respiratory droplets. The most common infection caused by *S. pyogenes* is an acute pharyngotonsilitis, but this organism has the ability to cause a broad spectrum of illness, from localized cellulitis to necrotizing pneumonia or fasciitis.

In children, a pharyngeal carrier state that elicits no immunologic response from the host is well described and can confound the accurate diagnosis of upper respiratory infection and/or confuse the interpretation of treatment directed at *S. pyogenes*. Untreated, *S. pyogenes* pharyngitis is usually a self-limiting, but painful disease. Treatment (usually penicillin G) is given primarily to prevent rheumatic fever, the most serious, non-suppurative complication of streptococcal pharyngitis. Treatment also prevents most of its relatively infrequent suppurative complications - otitis media, sinusitis, mastoiditis, cervical adenitis, or peritonsillar abscess.

Signs and Symptoms

While over 90% of pharyngitis illnesses in adults are due to viral agents, in children between the ages of three to twelve, *S. pyogenes* pharyngitis is common, with a late fall-wintertime peak. Classic complaints in a child are fever, headache, abdominal pain, and vomiting, with or without sore throat. On physical examination, tender cervical adenopathy, exudative tonsillitis, palatal petechiae, fetid breath, a white coated or red tongue, and sometimes a fine, erythematous, sandpaper-like (scarletiniform) rash, may be present. Signs typically associated with viral upper respiratory infection (e.g., coryza, cough, rhinorrhea) are absent.

S. pyogenes pharyngitis is distinctly uncommon in children less than three years old. Exudative tonsillitis, fever, and cervical adenopathy in this age group are more likely to be Epstein-Bar Virus infection (infectious mononucleosis). When streptococcal infection does occur in this group, it is more often a febrile syndrome of malaise, lymphadenopathy, and muco-purulent rhinorrhea, without pharyngitis. Scarlet fever results from infection with a *S. pyogenes* strain that produces an erythrogenic toxin. It, too, is uncommon in children less than three years of age.

Diagnosis of *S. pyogenes* pharyngitis is made by culture of the organism or by detecting *S. pyogenes* antigens by "rapid Strep test." The rapid tests have good specificity, meaning that if they are positive, the organism is present, but they lack sensitivity, that is, if the test is negative, it does not rule out the presence of the organism. Therefore, current recommendations for streptococcal pharyngitis testing in children are to perform rapid strep testing first, and if negative, to perform a throat culture. Current guidelines from the American Academy of Pediatrics recommend against testing for *S. pyogenes* in children with signs of upper respiratory tract infection to avoid the problems encountered with the *S. pyogenes* carrier state. In adults, because the incidence of streptococcal pharyngitis is very low, the recommendation is to perform rapid testing and decide on management based upon those results alone (Bisno et al., 2002).

Treatment

Penicillin G remains the drug of choice for treatment of streptococcal pharyngitis. Although first and second generation cephalosporins are more effective at eradicating the organism than penicillin, their ability to prevent rheumatic fever is not proven as it is for penicillin. For penicillin allergic individuals, erythromycin is the alternative treatment.

Breastfeeding and Group A Streptococcus

S. pyogenes pharyngitis is infrequent in children less than three years old. Mothers who contract the illness should seek treatment promptly as they may transmit the infection for about 24 hours after treatment begins. Efforts should be made to prevent transmission of the infection to the infant by limiting the infant's exposure to the mother's oral secretions. Good handwashing by the mother before contact with her infant is also prudent.

Summary

Streptococcal pharyngitis in infants less than three years old is uncommon. Mothers with streptococcal pharyngitis can breastfeed, but need to be aware that their oral/respiratory droplet secretions can transmit infection and that antibiotic treatment requires about 24 hours to decrease the risk of transmission.

Reference

Bisno AL, Gerber MA, Qwaltney JM, Jr, Kaplan RL, Schwartz RH, Infectious Disease Society of America. Practice guidelines for the diagnosis and management of group A streptococcal pharyngitis. Clin Infect Dis 25:113-125, 2002.

Group B Streptococcus (GBS)

Streptococcus agalactiae, the group B ß-hemolytic streptococcus (GBS), is a common colonizer of the healthy female genitourinary tract. Its acquisition by an infant during passage through a colonized birth canal can result in severe illness/sepsis in the infant during the newborn period. Two forms of GBS sepsis are recognized, "early onset" disease (presenting between zero to six days post partum) and "late onset" disease (presenting between seven days and three months postpartum). The clinical characteristics of the two forms are different: early onset is typically a sepsis/shock presentation, commonly accompanied by pneumonia and occasionally by meningitis, while late onset disease is typically meningitis. In late onset disease, occult bacteremia or focal disease (osteomyelitis, septic arthritis, cellulitis, adenitis) may accompany the meningitis. GBS is also a cause of mastitis (asymptomatic or symptomatic) in the lactating mother, and cases of GBS transmission from mother to infant via the milk are well documented.

Signs and Symptoms

Colonization of the female genitourinary tract is usually asymptomatic. Infection of the infant may be accompanied by lethargy, low body temperature, jaundice, poor feeding, apnea, or bradycardia. GBS infection in an infant is always a serious condition and is routinely treated with intravenous antibiotics.

It is now standard care to screen pregnant women for vaginal and rectal GBS carriage at 35-38 weeks gestation, and if colonized, to administer intrapartum chemoprophylaxis (antibiotic prophylaxis) starting at rupture of membranes or onset of labor. Additional indications for intrapartum antibiotic prophylaxis against GBS are:

- invasive GBS disease in a previous infant
- isolation of GBS from the urine anytime during pregnancy
- unknown maternal GBS status plus delivery at less than 37 weeks gestation, or ruptured membranes for >18 hours, or intrapartum maternal temperature >38.0 °C.

Treatment

Intrapartum chemoprophylaxis comprises either 2.5 million units of penicillin G intravenously every four hours (an alternative is ampicillin, 2 grams initially, then 1 gram every four hours intravenously). In penicillin allergic individuals, cefazolin, 2 grams initially followed by 1 gram IV every eight hours, is the preferred regimen.

Infants born to mothers who have received appropriate intrapartum chemoprophylaxis should not receive additional treatment for GBS unless they develop clinical illness compatible with invasive infection. Infants with invasive GBS infection are treated with intravenous antibiotics (usually treated initially with IV ampicillin plus an aminoglycoside), and once the organism is identified, penicillin G can be continued as treatment. Determination of whether meningitis is present should be done promptly as this diagnosis results in more prolonged courses of antibiotic treatment.

Breastfeeding and GBS Infection

Women colonized with GBS can breastfeed, but because of the intimate nature of nursing, the infant should be closely observed for signs of infection. Although GBS can be transmitted to the infant via breastmilk, with or without clinical signs of mastitis in the mother, this is an infrequent occurrence and should not cause great concern to the nursing mother who is colonized with GBS. It is reasonable and prudent for mothers with GBS colonization to be aware of this potential problem and to observe their infants for development of signs or symptoms suggestive of illness.

Summary

GBS colonization of the maternal genito-urinary tract is the usual route for neonatal acquisition. Intrapartum antibiotic chemoprophylaxis of colonized women significantly decreases the incidence of early onset invasive GBS disease in the infant. Transmission of GBS from mother to infant via breastmilk is described, but is an infrequent event.

Reference

Bingen E, Denamur E, Lambert-Zechovsky N, Aujard Y, Brahimi N, Geslin P, Elion J. Analysis of DNA restriction fragment length polymorphism extends the evidence for breast milk transmission of Streptococcus agalactiae late-onset neonatal infection. J Infect Dis 165:569-573, 1992.

Hand, Foot, and Mouth Disease (Coxsackievirus)

Hand, foot, and mouth disease is a clinical entity most commonly associated with enterovirus infection, usually either coxsackievirus A16 or enterovirus 71. Enteroviruses are a common cause of infantile illnesses characterized by rash, fever, and upper respiratory symptoms. Transmitted by both fecal-oral and respiratory routes, enteroviral illnesses are common in the summer and can spread quickly among children.

Signs and Symptoms

Hand, foot, and mouth disease is characterized by formation of blister-like lesions in the mouth and on the palms and soles (sometimes also on the buttock), often associated with fever, malaise, and cough. The fluid in the oral blisters contain the virus, hence oral secretions can transmit infection to other children. The oral blisters typically progress to ulcers, which are painful. The illness is self-limiting over several days, but because of the oral involvement, food intake may be decreased.

Treatment

No specific treatment is available for hand, foot, and mouth disease. Therefore, symptomatic care with attention to preventing dehydration is most important. Frozen juices, cold liquids, yogurt, or ice cream may be more acceptable than solid foods to the older infant and may need to be fed spoonful by spoonful. Use of over-the-counter analgesics, such as acetaminophen and ibuprofen, given before eating may help decrease the pain.

Breastfeeding and Coxsackievirus

No reported cases of transmission of hand, foot, and mouth disease from mother to infant or from infant to mother exist. Because of oral pain, breastfeeding may be rejected by the infant. In this instance, the mother should pump to maintain her milk supply.

Summary

Breastfeeding can continue without restriction during hand, foot, and mouth disease, but the infant may be transiently reluctant to nurse because of oral pain.

Reference

Sadeharju K, Knip M, Virtanen SNM, Savilahti E, Tauriainen S, Koskela P, Akerblom HK, Hyoty H, Finnish TRIGR study group. Maternal antibodies in breastmilk protect the child from enterovirus infections. Pediatrics 119:941-946, 2007.

Hepatitis A

Hepatitis A is an acute, self-limiting hepatitis associated with fecal-oral contamination. The virus that causes this disease is excreted in the stool of individuals with acute infection, hence, it is a disease associated with inadequate sanitation. Approximately 70% of cases in children less than six years old have no symptoms, while symptomatic infection occurs in about 70% of older children and adults. Chronic infection does not occur, and severe infection, while uncommon, can occur in individuals with underlying liver disease. Recognition of outbreaks because symptomatic disease develops in the parents or adult contacts of asymptomatically infected children is well described.

Signs and Symptoms

Clinical hepatitis A illness is characterized by fever, anorexia, malaise, nausea, and jaundice. By the time illness develops, fecal excretion of infectious virus has been ongoing for one to two weeks. Fecal excretion diminishes significantly by one week after onset of symptomatic illness, but more prolonged stool excretion can occur in infants and young children.

Diagnosis

The illness caused by hepatitis A virus is clinically indistinguishable from symptomatic hepatitis B or C infections. Diagnosis of acute or recent infection is made by detection of antibody (IgM type) against hepatitis A. Detection of IgG antibody against hepatitis A does not allow differentiation of acute, recent, or distant infection with hepatitis A virus.

Treatment

No specific treatment for hepatitis A is available. Active (vaccination) and passive (immune globulin administration) forms of immunoprophylaxis are available to prevent infection. Universal hepatitis A vaccination has recently been recommended for all children after twelve months of age. Pediatric and adult formulations of the vaccine are available, and both are given in a two- dose schedule (six to twelve months between doses). Immune globulin administration within two weeks of hepatitis A exposure is approximately 85% effective in preventing symptomatic infection, and immune globulin administration to travelers is recommended when areas where hepatitis A is endemic will be visited.

Breastfeeding and Hepatitis A

Hepatitis A is not transmitted via breastmilk. However, because hepatitis A is spread by the fecal-oral route, the intimacy of breastfeeding may create a situation that facilitates fecal-oral transmission. Because the greatest likelihood of virus transmission occurs when fecal excretion is highest (i.e., before symptoms of hepatitis A occur), good hand washing and personal hygiene by the breastfeeding mother are always recommended.

Summary

Hepatitis A is typically a self-limiting, acute disease transmitted via fecal-oral contamination. While no evidence for breastmilk transmission exists, transmission during the intimacy of breastfeeding could occur and would likely happen before onset of clinical symptoms in the mother. This reinforces the general recommendation that breastfeeding mothers exercise good hand washing and personal hygiene.

Reference

Stiehm ER, Keller MA. Breastmilk transmission of viral disease. Adv Nutr Res 10:105-122, 2001.

Hepatitis B

Hepatitis B is a DNA virus typically transmitted by contact with blood and/or body fluids. The illnesses it causes can range from symptomless illness to fulminant hepatitis with liver failure, and the duration of infection can vary from self-limiting to life-long. Perinatal acquisition is associated with development of chronic infection, and up to 25% of perinatally-acquired cases develop hepatocellular carcinoma or cirrhosis in adulthood.

Groups with increased risk for acquisition of hepatitis B include IV drug users, people with multiple heterosexual partners, homosexual men, healthcare workers who have contact with blood or body fluids, and the sexual partners of individuals with acute or chronic infection.

Signs and Symptoms

Hepatitis B infection is often asymptomatic. In individuals who develop symptoms, non-specific complaints, such as malaise, anorexia and nausea, may occur, or progressive specific signs of hepatitis with or without arthritis/arthralgia, macular rash, or thrombocytopenia may be prominent.

Fulminant, fatal hepatitis is uncommon, but can occur. Age at the time of acute infection is the major determinant of risk for developing chronic infection. Most (>90%) of infants acquiring infection perinatally develop chronic infection. Acquisition between one to five years of age decreases this risk to 25-50%, and acquisition in adulthood lowers it further to 6-10%.

Diagnosis

Hepatitis B cannot be differentiated from other types of acute hepatitis on the basis of clinical findings or routine laboratory testing. Specific blood testing for a panel of hepatitis B markers must be performed for diagnosis, and the patterns of the markers (i.e., present/absent) give insight into the stage of infection and whether the infection is acute or chronic.

Treatment

Hepatitis B is a disease better prevented than treated. Treatment of chronic infection with interferon-γ results in durable remission or cure in 20%-

40% of cases. Prevention is achieved with active and passive immunization approaches. Blood and body fluids from a patient with hepatitis B [i.e., their blood is (+) for hepatitis B surface antigen - HBsAg] are considered infectious, but if hepatitis B e antigen is present along with HBsAg, they are considered exquisitely infectious (tiny blood or body fluid exposures can transmit infection). This information can be important because it helps determine whether only active (hepatitis B vaccine) or active and passive (hepatitis B immunoglobulin - HBIG) immunoprophylaxis should be administered to contacts of a newly diagnosed individual with infection.

Hepatitis B vaccine is administered in a three or four dose series over six months depending upon patient factors. Universal pre-exposure vaccination is now recommended for all children starting between birth and two months of age, with the exception of infants born to mothers with hepatitis B. Because perinatal acquisition of hepatitis B by infants from their mothers is typically due to blood exposure at birth, infants born to HBSAg positive mothers should receive HBIg within twelve hours of delivery and begin their vaccination series immediately. Recommendations for hepatitis B testing after exposure and for administration of immunoprophylactic measures vary based on many factors: birth weight, types of exposure, patient age, and other risk factors. Therefore, seeking professional advice regarding transmission risk and prophylaxis options is usually appropriate.

Breastfeeding and Hepatitis B

Hepatitis B virus has been detected in human milk from mothers with infection, but epidemiologic data indicate breastfeeding does not significantly increase the risk of infection in infants of these mothers. In addition, infants of mothers with hepatitis B should have received both active and passive immunoprophylaxis starting at birth. Therefore, breastfeeding is not contraindicated in women with hepatitis B. The one caveat (because transmission occurs through blood or body fluid contact) is that should nipple injury or bleeding occur, it may be prudent to temporarily discontinue breastfeeding until healing occurs.

There are no data to suggest that either active or passive immunoprophylaxis is detrimental to the fetus/infant during pregnancy or lactation. Therefore, hepatitis B vaccination and HBIg administration are not contraindicated in either pregnancy or lactation.

Summary

Hepatitis B is transmitted through contact with blood or body fluids from infected individuals. Prevention of infection is much more effective than treatment. Screening of pregnant women for hepatitis B is necessary to allow appropriate immunoprophylaxis of infants born to mothers with hepatitis B. Breastfeeding is not contraindicated in hepatitis B, with appropriate consideration of preventing nursing infant contact with maternal blood.

Reference

Hill JB, Sheffield JS, Kim MJ, Alexamder JM, Sercely B, Wendel GD. Risk of hepatitis B transmission in breast fed infants of chronic hepatitis B carriers. Obstet Gynecol 99:1049-1052, 2002.

Hepatitis C (Non-A, Non-B Hepatitis)

The virus that causes hepatitis C is a RNA virus that is acquired primarily through contact with infected blood, either directly (e.g., transfusion) or indirectly (e.g., blood contaminated body fluids). Until recently when specific methods for testing units of blood for transfusion were developed, it was the most common cause of "post-transfusion hepatitis." As might be expected, rates of infection are highest in people with high or repeated direct exposure to blood or blood products. Estimates are that approximately 1-2% of pregnant women in the US are infected. The risk of perinatal transmission from an infected mother to her infant is about 5%, but this transmission only occurs in women who have hepatitis C RNA in their blood at the time of delivery.

Signs and Symptoms

Most hepatitis C infections are either asymptomatic or insidiously progressive. When symptoms of hepatitis C occur (anorexia, malaise, jaundice), they are clinically indistinguishable from hepatitis A or B. Persistent infection occurs in about 60-70% of adult cases, often without biochemical evidence of liver disease. In the US, hepatitis C infection is the leading reason for liver transplantation.

Diagnosis

Diagnosis is established by demonstrating presence of antibody against hepatitis C or by qualitative detection of hepatitis C RNA in the blood. If screening with a test for antibody is positive, it is repeated using a second generation Western blot test (Recombinant Immunoblot Assay-II, referred to as RIBA-II) to confirm the diagnosis. Testing for viral RNA is more prone to error than the antibody tests because specimen handling and the common phenomenon of intermittent presence of RNA in the blood of infected individuals impact test results and, consequently, their clinical usefulness.

Treatment

Several drug regimens using interferon-γ alone or in combination with other agents have been used to treat chronic hepatitis C infection in adults, but sustained responses to treatment are achieved in only 10-40% of cases. No vaccine or antibody immunoprophylaxis is available to prevent hepatitis C infection.

Breastfeeding and Hepatitis C

Maternal hepatitis C infection is not currently considered a contraindication to breastfeeding because transmission to the infant by this route has not been documented in mothers who are hepatitis C positive (and HIV negative). However, both antibodies against hepatitis C, as well as viral antigenic material, have been detected in milk from infected mothers, suggesting the theoretical possibility that infection could be transmitted by human milk. Therefore, the American Academy of Pediatrics recommends that the decision of a mother with hepatitis C infection to breastfeed should be based on informed discussion between the mother and her healthcare professional (American Academy of Pediatrics, 2006).

Summary

Hepatitis C is transmitted by infected human blood or body fluids contaminated by infected blood. Chronic infection is common and often leads to end-stage liver disease. Treatments for hepatitis C are moderately effective, and no preventative treatments are available. Hepatitis C virus can be shed in human milk, but no documented transmission of hepatitis C antibody (+) from infected women to their infants via breastmilk has occurred. Because a theoretical risk of transmission by milk exists, the decision whether or not to breastfeed is complex and should be made after informed discussion with the mother's healthcare provider.

Reference

American Academy of Pediatrics. Hepatitis C. In Pickering LK, Baker CJ, Long SS, McMillan JA, eds. Redbook: 2006 report of the Committee on Infectious Diseases, 27th edition. Elk Grove Village, IL: American Academy of Pediatrics, 2006: pp 355-359.

Herpes Simplex Virus Infection

Herpes simplex viruses 1 and 2 cause life-long infections in humans, with recurrent episodes of clinical illness. Herpes simplex virus 1 (HSV-1) is commonly associated with mouth (oropharyngeal) infections and HSV-2 is usually associated with genital infections, but either type can be isolated from any location and simultaneous infection with both types is possible. Genital HSV infection is a sexually transmitted disease. Oropharyngeal infection is usually transmitted by contact with infected secretions. For both oropharyngeal and genital infections in immunologically normal individuals, the first ("primary") episode of clinical disease is usually the most severe and longest lasting. Recurrences after clearance of the primary infection are the rule, (oropharyngeal recurrences are often called "fever blisters") and may be triggered by emotional or physiologic stress or for unknown reasons. Dissemination of HSV-1 or HSV-2 to distant body sites occurs infrequently, but can be a severe and damaging illness if the brain is involved (HSV encephalitis) or if dissemination occurs in an infant. Infants are particularly prone to severe disease. If they acquire their infection as a result of birth through a primary genital infection, attack rates for clinical illness approach 50%.

Recurrent HSV episodes occur because the virus establishes itself in a latent form in the nervous system following primary infection. The affected nerves usually are those that innervate the area of primary infection. After resolution of the primary infection, the virus remains latent in the nerve tissues without symptoms. When triggered to reactivate, the virus emerges from the nerves to cause skin manifestations in the same approximate area as the primary infection.

Signs and Symptoms

The typical sequence in a child or adult who develops either primary or recurrent localized HSV disease is initially burning/tingling in apparently normal skin where the outbreak will occur. This progresses to development of a blister or clusters of blisters that are tender. After the blisters open, they often form ulcers, which eventually scab and heal. For primary infections, the time course of this process is ten to fourteen days. In all forms, the blister fluid teems with infectious virus, and secretions from the area are infectious until the lesions are dry. Primary infections in the mouth and upper GI tract (herpetic gingivostomatitis) are most common in children between one and three years of age and can be so painful that oral intake and hydration become problems. Primary and recurrent genital infection is usually obvious in males, but may not be obvious in females because blisters on the vagina or cervix without skin lesions may go unnoticed. Unfortunately, once infected, genital shedding of HSV can occur without any obvious lesions, which can result in transmission of infection to uninfected sexual partners or to infants at birth without any obvious evidence of clinical disease in the index case.

Direct inoculation of HSV into the skin, with resulting infection, can occur after contact with an HSV lesion or contaminated instrument. This mechanism is likely responsible for breast HSV infection, scalp HSV infection at sites of fetal scalp blood sampling or scalp electrode placement, and transmission from a lip fever blister.

Diagnosis

The manifestations of HSV infection are often so characteristic that diagnosis, particularly of recurrent episodes, can be made clinically. In instances when a laboratory diagnosis is needed, culture of HSV from lesions or from mucosal surfaces or detection of HSV nucleic acid (DNA) by polymerase chain reaction (PCR) methods are used. In infants potentially exposed during birth, the sites usually cultured are moist skin folds, the umbilicus, oral/nasal mucosa, and rectum. Serologic diagnosis of HSV by detection of antibody against HSV can be helpful for classifying diseases as primary or recurrent, but is of little help for recognition/identification of HSV clinical illness.

In neonates, HSV infection can present without any evidence of cutaneous lesions, mimicking neonatal sepsis with fever and sometimes little else. With this clinical presentation, empiric antiviral and antibacterial treatments are often initiated together and continued until the cultures and PCR tests either establish a diagnosis or return negative.

Treatment

Antiviral agents active against HSV are available (acyclovir, valacyclovir) in intravenous, oral, and topical forms. The most effective method of treatment is intravenous administration because oral absorption of some agents is limited. Intravenous therapy is usually reserved for severe infections. Treatment does not eliminate infection - it speeds resolution of the current episode, but recurrences are not prevented.

The duration of intravenous treatment for neonatal HSV infection is usually 14 to 21 days depending on the type and severity of illness. Neonatal HSV infection is a dreaded condition because development of severe disease is common and devastating effects can occur even in the face of appropriate treatment with antiviral agents. It is a condition to avoid. Therefore, it is standard practice to deliver infants by cesarean section when women in labor have genital HSV lesions. This approach decreases the frequency of neonatal infection, but does not eliminate it because mother-to-infant transmission can occur in the absence of clinical findings (genital blisters) in the mother.

Breastfeeding and HSV Infection

Because of the intimacy of breastfeeding, a mother with clinical HSV infection presents a risk for transmission to the infant. This risk can be minimized if the mother understands how transmission occurs and exercises good hand washing and personal hygiene at all times, but particularly until the HSV lesions are dry. Kissing a newborn infant when a fever blister is present on or near the lips is inappropriate. HSV is probably not present in mother's milk in the absence of an HSV lesion on the nipple, areola, or the breast. Mother-to-infant transmission in the presence of a breast lesion has been described, as has transmission from infant-to-breast. HSV infection of the breast near to or on the areola or nipple is a contraindication to breastfeeding from that breast and probably feeding of expressed milk from that breast. If breastfeeding from the unaffected breast continues, care should be taken to prevent contact of infected fluids with the nursing infant. Once moist lesions are dry/scabbed, they are not considered to be infectious.

Summary

HSV infection is usually a limited illness in a lactating mother, but usually a serious illness in the newborn infant. HSV infection in a breastfeeding mother poses variable degrees of risk for transmission to the infant depending on the site of infection and whether contact of infected fluids with the infant occurs. HSV infection of the breast near to or on the areola or nipple is a contraindication to breastfeeding from that breast. Once moist HSV lesions are dry/scabbed, they are not considered infectious.

References

Amir J, Harel L, Smetana Z, Varsano I. The natural history of primary herpes simplex type 1 gingivostomatitis in children. Pediatr Dermatol 16:259-263, 1999.

Schreiner RL, Kleiman MB, Gresham EL. Maternal oral herpes: isolation policy. Pediatrics 63:247-249, 1979.

Sealander JY, Kerr CP. Herpes simplex of the nipple: infant-to-mother transmission. Am Fam Physician 39:111-113, 1989.

Sullivam-Bolyai JZ, Fife KH, Jacobs RF, Miller Z, Corey L. Disseminated neonatal herpes simplex virus type 1 from a maternal breast lesion. Pediatrics 71:455-457, 1983.

Human Immunodeficiency Virus (HIV/AIDS)

Infection with human immunodeficiency virus (HIV) results in life-long infection, which, if left untreated, causes progressive loss of cellular immunity systems, which leads to life-threatening/life-ending infections. Two types of HIV are recognized: HIV-1 and HIV-2. HIV-1 causes more than 90% of infections worldwide, while pockets of HIV-2 infection are known in East Africa, parts of the Caribbean, and in Central America. HIV-1 and HIV-2 are transmitted by contact with infected body fluids. Sexual contact, intravenous drug use, and, historically, contact with blood or blood products, are the major routes of transmission. Vertical transmission from mother to infant during pregnancy, at birth, or postpartum via breastmilk occurs.

Signs and Symptoms

Acute infection with HIV results in a mild systemic illness with associated lymphadenopathy. After resolution of these symptoms, HIV infection is largely silent until it produces significant immunodeficiency via depletion of T-cells. At that point, the risk of opportunistic infection increases significantly, and when these occur, testing for an underlying HIV infection is usually done as part of the diagnostic evaluation. *In utero* infection can have no clinical findings at birth, or may result in low birth weight or generalized lymphadenopathy that is first appreciated immediately after birth.

Diagnosis

HIV infection can be identified by antibody-based or nucleic acid detection methods. Screening tests for HIV infection depend on detection of antibody against a specific HIV protein called p24. If anti-p24 is detected, a second test (HIV western blot test) is performed which determines whether antibody against other HIV components are present. If they are, HIV infection is confirmed. In infants born to HIV infected mothers, transplacental passage of maternal antibody (without actual infection of the fetus/infant) can result in (+) p24 and HIV western blot tests at birth, giving these tests limited usefulness for diagnosis of neonatal HIV infection. Therefore, a polymerase chain reaction (PCR) test for HIV-DNA is performed on at risk infants several days after birth and is repeated at two and four months of age.

For management of HIV infected individuals, determination of the "viral load" and the number of T-lymphocytes in the blood are used to assess effectiveness of treatment. Viral load is measured using a PCR HIV-RNA test.

Treatment

Treatment and management of adult and pediatric HIV infection is a complex, ongoing process that requires guidance by an experienced physician. Three large classes of anti-HIV medications, nucleoside agents, non-nucleoside agents, and protease inhibitors are available alone and in combinations that are selected based upon patient status, HIV resistance, prior treatment history, side effects, drug interactions, and toxicities. HIV infection without treatment results in progressive loss of immunity, opportunistic infection, and death. HIV infection with treatment results in life-long infection and risks of treatment-related toxicities. Avoidance of HIV infection remains the best approach to its management.

Breastfeeding and HIV Infection

Despite the fact that human milk contains components that could be protective against HIV transmission, epidemiologic data clearly indicate that HIV transmission through breastfeeding occurs. Therefore, the recommendations of the World Health Organization and the American Academy of Pediatrics are largely the same: the HIV (+) mother should avoid breastfeeding when safe feeding alternatives are available. In the under-developed world, safe feeding alternatives may not always be available, and so in some instances, breastfeeding by an HIV-infected mother may be the only reasonable option. Shorter duration and exclusive breastfeeding by HIV infected mothers has lower risks of transmission than longer duration breastfeeding, feeding milk from multiple mothers, or mixed feeding. When breastfeeding by an HIV-infected mother is necessary, it should be exclusive breastfeeding and for the shortest possible period.

Summary

Maternal HIV infection is a contraindication to breastfeeding when safe feeding alternatives are readily available. In the situation where they are not, the decision to breastfeed should be based on informed discussion between the HIV-infected mother and her healthcare provider, and exclusive breastfeeding for as short a duration as possible should be used to minimize the risks of HIV transmission as much as possible.

Reference

Fowler MG, Lampe MA, Jamieson DJ, Kourtis AP, Rogers MF. Reducing the risk of mother-to-child human immunodeficiency virus transmission: past successes, current progress and challenges, and future directions. Am J Obstet Gynecol 197 (3 suppl) S3-9, 2007.

Influenza

Influenza is an acute respiratory infection that is the most important cause of wintertime respiratory illness world wide. It is caused by influenza virus and spreads through the population every year. The severity of the annual influenza outbreak varies from year to year, depending upon how closely the current year's strain is related to the previous year's strains and the time of onset of the outbreak. When strains are very different or the outbreak starts in the fall rather than winter, the influenza outbreak is usually more severe. Three types of influenza are recognized - influenza A, B, and C. Influenza A and B are the prominent pathogens in humans. Many species can be infected by influenza, but the ability of strains to cross species lines is somewhat limited. When it does occur, a very different strain often emerges, resulting in a significant increase in the severity of the influenza season.

Influenza is usually transmitted from person to person by respiratory droplets aerosolized by the coughing of a person infected with influenza. The cough of influenza can last for weeks, although infectivity usually declines after five to seven days. The major complications of influenza are bacterial pneumonia, sinusitis, and in children, otitis media.

Signs and Symptoms

Influenza usually begins acutely, over several hours, during which time the person goes from feeling well to feeling ill. Tracheitis is the first clinical manifestation of influenza, followed shortly thereafter by cough, coryza, fever, chills, headache, malaise, nasal congestion, and myalgia. The illness usually lasts five to seven days, but the hacking cough can persist beyond all other symptoms.

Treatment

Two types of medications are available for treatment of influenza. Amantadine and rimantidine are similar drugs that block uncoating of (only) influenza A after it enters a target cell. Zanamivir and oseltamivir represent the other type of anti-influenza drug and are agents that block neuraminidase activity of both influenza A and B (CDC, 2005). Both types of drugs require rapid, precise diagnosis of influenza, as well as identification of the type of influenza, because to be effective, they need to be started within 48 hours of the onset of symptoms. Tests that allow rapid identification and typing of influenza viruses have been clinically available for only about five years.

Prevention of influenza through annual immunization is a more effective approach to control than treatment. An inactivated virus vaccine (the "flu shot") has been available for several decades, and a temperature adapted live virus vaccine that is administered into the nose has become available in the past four years.

Inactivated influenza vaccines are prepared every year, and contain three strains of killed influenza virus (usually two A strains and one B strain). The choice of strains is based upon the likely strains that will be circulating in the upcoming influenza season, and the choices are not always perfect. The temperature adapted vaccine is also produced annually to match the influenza strains expected to be in circulation the next year.

Influenza vaccination is now recommended for many groups (CDC, 2005), including:

- Persons 50 years and older
- Occupants of nursing homes and chronic care facilities
- Adults and children requiring follow-up for chronic metabolic disease
- Adults and children with conditions that can compromise respiratory function
- Children six months to 18 years on chronic aspirin therapy
- Women who will be pregnant during influenza season
- Children six to 23 months of age
- Healthcare workers
- Persons who can transmit influenza to those at high risk for infection.

Breastfeeding and Influenza Medications

Little information on the use of influenza treatment medications in lactating women is available. Amantadine, rimantidine, and oseltamivir are approved for use in children one year and older. The influenza vaccination is safe for breastfeeding mothers (CDC, 2005).

Breastfeeding and Influenza

The highest risk period for transmission of influenza is the 24 hours before appearance of symptoms. Thus, by the time the breastfeeding mother suspects she has influenza, her infant has already had significant exposure. Because breastfeeding will likely provide some protection against development of infection in the infant, breastfeeding should continue. With the mother ill, she needs to get rest and to remain well hydrated. She should be comfortable with feeding the baby in bed with her, but must also ensure the infant's safety when she sleeps (i.e., she and the infant sleep in close proximity such that there is no threat of "roll-over" injury). Throughout her illness, the mother should practice good hand washing and avoid coughing or sneezing directly onto the infant, but in reality, the infant is at high risk for developing infection.

Should a breastfeeding mother develop influenza, both parents should be observant for signs of illness in their infant. In small children, influenza can present as a "cold" or as a high fever with respiratory illness. If concerned, parents should contact their infant's physician, particularly if maintaining the infant's hydration becomes a concern, if fever becomes high and persistent, or if the illness is prolonged. Infants with influenza should continue to breastfeed.

Summary
The mother with influenza can breastfeed, as can the infant with influenza.

References
CDC. Prevention and control of influenza. Recommendations of the Advisory Committee on Immunization Practices. MMWR (July 29, 2005) 54 (No RR-8).

Jaundice, Breastmilk

Jaundice associated with breastfeeding is two clinical entities: one occurs early in life (during the first week) and is an accentuation of hyperbilirubinemia of the newborn. This is called "**breastfeeding jaundice.**" The other occurs later (seven to fifteen days of life) as persistence of hyperbilirubinemia of the newborn and is called "**breastmilk jaundice.**" One author has said that "breastfeeding jaundice" is more accurately referred to as "breast nonfeeding jaundice" (Gartner, 2001) because it develops as a result of inadequate volumes of breastmilk consumed by the infant (AAP, 2004), resulting in relative dehydration. "Breastmilk jaundice" is less well understood and may be multi-factorial. Its occurrence is related in part to the action of an unknown component in breastmilk that enhances reabsorption of unconjugated bilirubin from the bowel after it has been excreted in the bile. In addition, several types of mutations in specific bilirubin metabolism genes have been implicated (Maruo et al., 2000; Monaghan et al., 1999) as contributing to "breastmilk jaundice." Regardless of the cause of the jaundice, the clinical implications of severe elevations in unconjugated bilirubin are the same as described below for neonatal jaundice.

Signs and Symptoms
Infants who develop "breastfeeding jaundice" are at increased risk for poor weight gain and hypernatremia (Tarcan et al., 2005) because their oral intake is inadequate. Infants who develop "breastmilk jaundice" are typically doing

well, thriving, gaining weight appropriately, passing stools normally, and feeding well. They have no other manifestations other than jaundice.

Diagnosis

Diagnosis is based on breastfeeding history, time of appearance, and measurement of the blood bilirubin levels.

Treatment

The usual management of breastfeeding jaundice is to increase the infant's breastmilk consumption by feeding eight to twelve times/day for the first several days. If this cannot be done, then oral supplementation with infant formula, electrolyte solution, or water, or intravenous fluid administration may be necessary. In extreme situations, intravenous hydration is used.

The usual management of "breastmilk jaundice" is transient discontinuation of breastfeeding over 12 to 24 hours, with substitution of infant formula. This sort of interruption of breastfeeding usually results in a prompt decline in bilirubin levels, after which breastfeeding can be resumed. With resumption, bilirubin levels may again rise, then begin a slow decline. The most difficult question is at what level of hyperbilirubinemia should breastfeeding be interrupted if the infant is otherwise healthy. There is no precise, universally accepted answer to this question: it is a clinical judgment. If a decision to interrupt breastfeeding is made, the mother should be encouraged to pump to maintain her milk production, so that breastfeeding can be re-initiated promptly after the bilirubin level falls.

Breastfeeding and Breastmilk Jaundice

Usually after discontinuation of breastfeeding, the elevated bilirubin levels of Breastmilk Jaundice decline promptly. Thereafter, breastfeeding can be resumed under the guidance of a clinician, usually with continued monitoring of bilirubin levels.

Summary

Breastmilk jaundice is likely to be due to a poorly characterized component in breastmilk that enhances reabsorption of bilirubin from the bowel into the circulation. Once diagnosis has been established, breastfeeding can continue with monitoring of bilirubin levels.

References

American Academy of Pediatrics Subcommittee on Hyperbilirubinemia. Management of hyperbilirubinemia in the newborn infant 35 or more weeks of gestation. Pediatrics 114:297-316, 2004.

Gartner LM. Breastfeeding and jaundice. J Perinatol 21 Suppl 1:S25-S29, 2001.

Maruo Y, Nishizawa K, Sato H, Sawa H, Shimada M. Prolonged unconjugated hyperbilirubinemia associated with breast milk and mutations of the bilirubin uridine diphosphate-glucuronosyltransferase gene. Pediatrics 106:e59, 2000. (http://www.pediatrics.org/cgi/content/full/106/5/e59).

Monaghan G, McLellen A, McGeehan A, Li Volti S, Mollica F, Salemi I, et al. Gilbert's syndrome is a contributory factor in prolonged unconjugated hyperbilirubinemia of the newborn. J Pediatr 134:441-446, 1999.

Tarcan A, Yiker F, Vatandas NS, Haberal A, Gurakan B. Weight loss and hypernatremia in breast-fed babies: frequency in neonates with non-hemolytic jaundice. J Paediatr Child Health 41:484-487, 2005.

Jaundice, Neonatal (Hyperbilirubinemia of the Newborn)

At birth, many infants do not have fully matured liver functions that clear bilirubin from their blood. As a result, "neonatal jaundice" or "physiologic jaundice of the newborn" is a common condition; it usually resolves by two to three weeks of age because of liver maturation.

When babies develop *in utero*, their oxygen supply is fully dependent on the placental blood supply, and they have high concentrations of red blood cells in their circulation to capture and transport oxygen efficiently to their developing tissues. When babies begin to breathe air on their own at birth, they no longer need these high concentrations of red cells and spontaneously decrease their red blood cell production to allow the red cell concentration in their blood to fall toward normal levels. As old red blood cells are removed from the circulation, they release hemoglobin (the protein that carries oxygen), which is converted to bilirubin. Usually, the bilirubin is chemically modified ("conjugated") in the liver to allow its excretion into the stool via the bile. Because babies often have not fully matured their liver mechanism to conjugate bilirubin by the time they are born, persistence of unconjugated bilirubin in the blood of the neonate ("neonatal jaundice") is a common occurrence. The difficulty is that if unconjugated bilirubin rises to high levels, there is a toxic effect on parts of the brain, resulting in a severe neurological condition called "acute bilirubin encephalopathy." Therefore, pediatricians closely monitor the levels of bilirubin in neonatal jaundice, following the amounts of unconjugated and conjugated forms and how they change over time in the blood of newborn infants.

Conditions in the mother or infant that result in more rapid destruction of red blood cells make neonatal jaundice more severe, and therefore, more serious. Blood group incompatability between infant and mother (e.g., Rh or ABO incompatability) or antibody-mediated hemolytic anemia in the mother need to be identified either pre-partum or rapidly in the peripartum period to allow appropriate diagnosis and expectant management.

While neonatal/physiologic jaundice is common in normal infants, it is not the only cause of jaundice in the neonate. A long list of conditions, some severe, can cause jaundice during this time. Whether to pursue other causes for jaundice depends on the severity, progression, persistence, and biochemical characteristics of the infant's jaundice.

Signs and Symptoms

Neonatal jaundice presents as yellow-orange discoloration of the skin called ("jaundice"). Color change in the whites of the eyes is often the first change noticed by the parents. Urine color can change to deeper orange-yellow, and if shaken, the urine foam is yellow-orange instead of white. Usually no other symptoms are present.

Diagnosis

Jaundice can be recognized by observation, but the magnitude of jaundice/ hyperbilirubinemia requires measurement of blood bilirubin levels. These measurements may include total bilirubin levels or may divide the total bilirubin into conjugated and unconjugated fractions. Early on, neonatal jaundice is all due to unconjugated bilirubin, but as the infant's liver function matures, a conjugated bilirubin component appears as the total bilirubin level falls. Appearance of a conjugated bilirubin fraction usually indicates the beginning of the liver maturation needed to resolve neonatal jaundice.

Treatment

The approach to treatment depends on how quickly after birth jaundice appears and how fast the bilirubin level rises (AAP, 2004). If jaundice is mild and the bilirubin is not rising rapidly, patience and maintaining the infant's hydration is the usual approach. Because the blood bilirubin concentration depends on the infant's hydration level to a significant degree (dehydration raises the blood bilirubin concentration), maintaining hydration through frequent (eight to twelve feeds/day) breastfeeding is the simple approach.

If the bilirubin level dictates a more aggressive approach, phototherapy may be used. In the 1800s, it was noted that infants near nursery windows did not develop jaundice the way other infants did. Two hundred years later, it is known that specific blue wavelengths of light result in photodegradation of bilirubin. If bilirubin levels are rising, but are not acutely dangerous or if medical conditions are present that predict subsequent severe rises in bilirubin, application of phototherapy using "bili-lights" therapeutically or prophylactically is standard practice. In the past, phototherapy had to be administered as an inpatient, but novel and effective methods for home phototherapy are now available. In cases where bilirubin levels are acutely and dangerously high, two volume exchange transfusion (replacing twice the infants blood volume with transfused blood by repeated cycles of removing blood and replacing it by transfusion) may be necessary to lower the blood bilirubin level.

Breastfeeding and Neonatal Jaundice

If breastfeeding does not supply the infant with adequate amounts of water, it can worsen neonatal jaundice by creating a state of relative dehydration. The solution to this is to ensure eight to twelve feeds at the breast per day for the first several days, which provides both the opportunity for the infant to take in adequate amounts of fluid and stimulation to increase the mother's milk supply.

Summary

Neonatal jaundice is a common condition that results from immaturity of the infant's liver. With liver maturation, the condition resolves. Breastfeeding eight to twelve times a day for the first several days postpartum is recommended to minimize the impact of neonatal jaundice by both preventing relative dehydration in the infant and stimulating maternal milk production.

References

American Academy of Pediatrics Subcommittee on Hyperbilirubinemia. Management of hyperbilirubinemia in the newborn infant 35 or more weeks of gestation. Pediatrics 114:297-316, 2004.

Mastitis & Breast Abscess

Mastitis, inflammation of the breast, is a common problem during lactation, particularly in first-time mothers. It is reportedly the second most common reason given by mothers for discontinuing breastfeeding.

The structure of the breast as it relates to milk production is important in understanding the development of mastitis. Milk is produced in the alveolae of the breast (small clusters of milk producing chambers) and then is passed into the milk ducts and lacteals (tubular structures just below the areola) to the nipple. When milk is not emptied from the breast by regular nursing or expression, it builds up in the alveolar ducts and lacteals, and distends them. If these structures distended by milk cross over other milk ducts or lacteals, their distention can put pressure on neighboring structures and cause them to close/collapse. This obstruction can produce a type of milk flow grid lock that is called "milk stasis." If the milk stasis is not relieved, continued milk production results in further distention and further milk flow obstruction, resulting in increasing local inflammation ("plugged ducts"). Should bacteria enter the breast through the lacteals and progress to the distended areas, they can cause infection in the pooled milk which greatly increases the local inflammation to produce "mastitis." If the mastitis is not treated or relieved, the infection can progress to the point a "breast abscess" develops.

Not surprisingly, the factors that are associated with development of the plugged duct-mastitis-breast abscess continuum include: being in the first four months of lactation, having breast engorgement, missing feedings, not emptying the breast completely, wearing breast support garments that put pressure on the breast in discrete areas and result in obstruction of milk flow, and having maternal stress/fatigue.

The organisms commonly isolated from mastitis milk include *Staphylococcus aureus*, coagulase-negative staphylococci, and various types of streptococci. Of these, the most pathogenic is *Staphylococcus aureus*.

This organism tends to cause soft tissue infections and abscess diseases. Methicillin-susceptible *Staphylococcus aureus* (MSSA) strains have a long association with mastitis in lactating women. More recently, strains of methicillin-resistant *Staphylococcus aureus* (MRSA) have become more common as a cause of mastitis and perinatal infections in both mothers and infants (Saiman et al., 2003; Reddy et al., 2007; Fortunov et al., 2007). Nasal carriage of MSSA by an infant is associated with development of MSSA mastitis in the mother (Amir et al., 2006), and presumably the same applies for MRSA carriage. The potential for transmission of either MSSA or MRSA to an infant via breastfeeding has also been demonstrated in multiple instances (Kawada et al., 2003; Gastelum et al., 2005).

Signs and Symptoms

Local breast tenderness (milk stasis) that progresses to redness, warmth, swelling, and pain (plugged ducts), with subsequent development of fever and malaise usually indicates mastitis. Because there is often an anatomical component (the grid lock effect) to development of mastitis, if mastitis recurs, development in the same region of the breast is common.

Treatment

How the plugged duct mastitis breast abscess process is treated depends on the stage at which it is recognized. Since the problem is initiated by ineffective drainage of milk, the approach usually applied to milk stasis is local heat and massage of the affected area to try to get the pooled milk to drain. Nursing more frequently on the affected side is commonly used because the infant is much more efficient at milk removal than manual expression or breast pumping. If mastitis is present, treatment usually involves more frequent feeding to enhance drainage, plus treatment with oral antibiotics directed against *Staphylococcus aureus*. If breast abscess develops, the infant should not be fed from the affected side (breast abscess rupture while feeding can cause so much milk contamination that the infant becomes ill). Sonography-guided needle aspiration of the abscess or surgical drainage may be necessary, usually accompanied by antibiotic therapy.

Breastfeeding and Mastitis Medications

Antibiotics administered to the mother frequently pass in small amounts to the nursing infant. Usually, the amounts of antibiotic passed are so small that they do not affect the infant or interfere with the accuracy of cultures taken on the infant.

Breastfeeding and Mastitis/Breast Abscess

As a major component of treatment for mastitis is effective drainage of milk from the affected breast, and the nursing infant is by far the most effective method for draining the breast, nursing at increased frequency from the breast with mastitis is a long standing treatment recommendation. Breastfeeding may continue with no restrictions on the unaffected breast. Should a breast abscess develop, breastfeeding can resume 24 hours after onset of treatment with antibiotics if the abscess has not drained into the milk, or 24 hours following surgical drainage. Milk collected during the 24 hour period from the affected breast should be discarded.

Summary

Milk stasis, plugged milk ducts, mastitis, and breast abscess are a continuum of clinical conditions related to ineffective drainage of milk from the breast. Predisposing factors include engorgement, irregular feeding schedules, tight-fitting clothing, and breastfeeding inexperience. The nursing infant is the most effective method for removing milk from the breast and plays an important role in preventing and treating this continuum of conditions.

References

Amir LH, Garland SM, Lumley J. A case-control study of mastitis: nasal carriage of Staphylococcus aureus. BMC Fam Pract 7:57, 2006.

Fortunov RM, Hulten KG, Hammerman WA, et al. Evaluation and treatment of community-acquired Staphylococcus aureus infections in term and late pre-term previously healthy neonates. Pediatrics 120:937-945, 2007.

Gastelum DT, Dassey D, Mascola L, Yasuda LM. Transmission of community-associated methicillin-resistant Staphylococcus aureus from breast milk in the neonatal intensive care unit. Pediatr Infect Dis J 24:1122-1124, 2005.

Kawada M, Okuzumi S, Sugishita C. Transmission of Staphylococcus aureus between healthy, lactating mothers and their infants by breastfeeding. J Hum Lact 19:411-417, 2003.

Reddy P, Qi C, Zembower T, et al. Postpartum mastitis and community-acquired methicillin-resistant Staphylococcus aureus. Emerg Infect Dis 13:290-301, 2007.

Saiman L, O'Keefe M, Graham PL, et al. Hospital transmission of community-acquired methicillin-resistant Staphylococcus aureus among post-partum women. Clin Infect Dis 37:1313-1319, 2003.

Multiple Sclerosis

Multiple sclerosis (MS) is a progressive, inflammatory neurologic disease of unknown cause that affects about 1 in 1000 individuals in western countries. It is suspected of being an autoimmune disease (the result of the body immunologically attacking itself), and it usually begins in early adulthood. Women are affected more commonly than men, making the impact of MS on pregnancy and breastfeeding a serious consideration.

Signs and Symptoms:

Most frequently, MS is a disease that flares, that is, it has remissions (spontaneous improvements) and relapses (worsening symptoms). In fewer cases (15%), it is progressive. Because the inflammatory process and demyelination in the central nervous system (the brain and spinal cord) characteristic of MS can occur in any location, the signs and symptoms of this illness can be extremely variable. Changes in bowel or bladder function, decreased cognitive function, loss of coordination, strength, or balance, depression or emotional changes, numbness or tingling, diminished vision, and pain or development of spasticity can all be manifestations of MS. As a result, the criteria for diagnosis are relatively broad: evidence of disease in at least two different areas of the central nervous system and at least two flares of disease. MS is often suspected before these diagnostic criteria are met, and in some instances, testing by magnetic resonance imaging of the central nervous system, by examination of the cerebrospinal fluid, or by evoked brain potential measurements is done.

Pregnancy is a time of "immunologic truce" between the mother and the fetus she is carrying. The mother changes her body's defenses to avoid attacking the fetus as a "foreign tissue," and the fetus does not develop strong defenses while it is being carried by the mother to prevent the fetus from attacking the mother as a "foreign tissue." As such, many autoimmune diseases in women are known to subside during pregnancy, presumably because of the "truce," and after delivery, they reappear in the mother. The same is true for MS. MS relapses may decrease during pregnancy and then appear to increase in the first three months after pregnancy before returning to the "pre-pregnancy" relapse rate (Confavreux et al., 1998). There is no evidence that children born to women with MS are in any way physically or mentally affected by their mothers having MS while they were pregnant with them (Lorenzi & Ford, 2002).

Treatment

There is no cure for MS. Treatments to decrease the frequency/intensity of flares and/or slow progression of MS are an active area of clinical research, and at present, immunomodulatory (e.g., interferon-ß), immunosuppressive, and/or anti-inflammatory (corticosteroids) treatments are used. Continuing corticosteroid treatment during pregnancy and lactation poses little-to-no risk to the fetus and nursing infant. However, at present, use of immunomodulatory or immunosuppressive agents during pregnancy and lactation is not advised (Lorenzi & Ford, 2002) because of uncertainty about their safety for the fetus and nursing infant. In all cases, the characteristics of the woman's MS (its severity, its rate of progression, and frequency of relapses) must be considered and discussed between the mother and her physician to arrive at an individualized plan for her treatments, their compatibility with pregnancy, and their effects post-partum and during lactation.

Breastfeeding and Multiple Sclerosis

Multiple sclerosis is not a contraindication to breastfeeding. The immunomodulatory and immunosuppressive drugs used to treat and control its relapses can be potentially toxic for the nursing infant. Corticosteroid therapy is not a threat to the nursing infant.

Summary

Multiple sclerosis is a disease that occurs in women of reproductive age. Its severity and frequency of relapses appear to lessen during pregnancy, and then return after delivery of the infant. Immunomodulatory and immunosuppressive medications used to treat MS are not presently considered compatible with breastfeeding.

References

Confavreux C, Hutchinson M, Hours MM, Cortinovis-Tourniaire P, Moreau T. Rates of pregnancy-related relapse in multiple sclerosis. N Engl J Med 339:285-291, 1998.

Lorenzi AR, Ford HL. Multiple sclerosis and pregnancy. Postgrad Med J 78:460-464, 2002.

Neural Tube Defects

During intrauterine development of the fetus, the development of the structure that will become the brain and spinal cord, called the "neural tube," begins about day 18. It normally achieves a tube-like structure by day 23-28 through a process that brings its opposing edges together, called neural tube closure. Failure of the developmental process of neural tube closure produces defects of varying severity, depending on where and how extensive the failure to close is. While the causes for neural tube defects are not fully understood, it is known that after such a defect occurs in a child, the risk of recurrence in a subsequent child is about 3-4%; with two affected children, the risk rises to 10%. At present, the occurrence rates for neural tube malformations is less than 1 per 1000 live births. Maternal supplementation with folic acid significantly decreases the incidence of these defects.

Characteristics

Anencephaly: This is a severe and usually lethal malformation that results in failure of development of the entire brain. The bones of the upper skull are usually absent, as are major components of the brain: cerebral hemispheres, brainstem, and basal ganglia. An infant born with anencephaly is usually unable to develop, and death shortly after birth is typical.

Encephalocele: In this condition, the neural tube defect is more localized than in anencephaly, resulting in a gap in the skull structure and herniation of some part of the brain through the gap. The size of the gap and degree of brain herniation crucially impact prognosis. For all but the smallest defects, infant survival is usually short or severe mental retardation develops. In some rare instances, surgery can improve the prognosis somewhat.

Spina bifida: In this condition, the defect occurs at the opposite end of the neural tube compared to those that cause anencephaly or encephalocele. This condition is the most commonly seen of neural tube defects, and produces a defect in the structure of the spine, spinal cord, and spinal canal. In all instances, the tissues of the spinal cord "balloon" through a defect in the spine, but the precise name of the condition depends on the types of spinal tissues involved. If only the meninges (fine membranes that surround the spinal cord) are involved, the precise term is "meningocele." If the spinal cord without the meninges is involved, it is termed a "myelocele." If both are involved, the term(s) are "meningomyelocele" or "myelomeningocele."

Involvement of both cord and meninges occurs in about 80% of cases. The location of the defect can vary. About 70% of cases are in the lumbar or lumbosacral spine (the low back). Association of hydrocephalus (water on the brain) with spina bifida is common (about 75%). The ballooning of the meninges/cord in spina bifida usually causes damage to it where it balloons, with resulting paralysis below the injury. Thus, the level on the spine where the defect occurs predicts the severity and extent of paralysis. The legs are typically affected, but if the spinal defect occurs above the low back, more extensive loss of nerve function can occur. Because normal intrauterine development of bones and muscles depends on normal nerve function in the developing tissues, orthopedic deformities in the paralyzed tissues are common. Other complications that can be associated with spina bifida are abnormal brain structure, inadequate bladder control, precocious puberty, growth hormone deficiency, incontinence, or chronic constipation.

The size and location of the spine defect in spina bifida is important, both for its recognition and symptoms. "Spina bifida occulta" is the condition where the spinal defect is such that no ballooning of the cord or meninges can be observed externally. Instead, either no evidence, a tuft of hair, a dimple, or unusual pigmentation at the site of the deep defect is the only hint at birth that there is a deeper problem. These findings at birth usually trigger further investigation, but if no outward sign is present, this condition can be missed initially. As time progresses, however, this condition is often associated with delay in walking, low back or leg pain, or progressive abnormalities of the leg or foot, recognition of which leads to its diagnosis.

Treatment

The child with recognized spina bifida will usually have surgerical repair within 24 hours of birth. The surgery cannot undo damage that has already occurred, but it can minimize further damage, preserve existing nerve function, and decrease the risk of central nervous system infection. Subsequent surgeries as the child grows are common to repair orthopedic deformities and/or improve residual function in the affected tissues. Medical management of children with spina bifida has improved greatly over time, but they still require special efforts to ensure their mobility through the use of crutches, braces, and wheelchairs. Ongoing observation and early intervention for physical, emotional, psychological, or neurological changes as the child grows optimize their prognosis.

As the damage to the spinal cord has already occurred by the time a child with spina bifida is born, prevention of the malformation is a much better strategy than treatment. Consumption of adequate amounts of folic acid for at least three months pre-conception and during the first month of pregnancy is epidemiologically associated with a 50-72% lower risk of having an infant with a neural tube defect. This is why it is recommended for women of child-bearing age to consume at least 0.4 mg of folic acid/day. Folic acid is prevalent in dark green, leafy vegetables and is added to certain foods, such as enriched breads, pastas, rice, and cereals by their manufacturers.

Prenatal Diagnosis

Most neural tube defects are recognized at birth, but identification of their presence *in utero* can sometimes be achieved by measuring the α fetoprotein (AFP) level in the mother's blood early in pregnancy. In a fetus with a neural tube defect, AFP can leak through the defect into the amniotic fluid and then absorption into the maternal blood results in elevated AFP levels in the mother. If an elevated maternal blood AFP level is found between weeks 15-18 of gestation, a fetal ultrasound and sometimes direct sampling of the amniotic fluid (to measure its AFP level) are performed to determine whether a defect is present or not.

Breastfeeding and Neural Tube Defects

The infant with a neural tube defect can be fed human milk. Even if an infant is terminally ill due to a severe defect, the mother may desire to provide milk for her dying infant. Such wishes should not be disregarded. The medical impact of this action may be nil, but the psychological and social impact may be far reaching.

For the infant with a better long-term prognosis for growth and development, breastfeeding should be considered. The rooting and sucking reflexes are basic, and as long as coordinated and effective swallowing is present, infants with neural tube defects may be no different than other infants when it comes to breastfeeding. The challenges to appropriate positioning for breastfeeding that come from early corrective surgery - need to lay flat with minimal/no spine flexion, may require a more creative approach. The mother may have to bring the breast/nipple to the baby, rather than depending on the infant to find and latch itself. Some experts suggest this is best done with the mother in bed, the infant lying beside her, feeding in a side-lying position. Alternatively, placing the infant on a stiff surface, placing the infant/surface combination in the mother's lap, and then "free-lancing" to find a position that will get the nipple into the infant's mouth (creativity may be crucial) may result in success. Alternatively, expressed milk can be used until post-operative restrictions are lifted and the infant can be more easily positioned. While these approaches obviously require additional efforts on the part of many people, they are worth the effort because breastfeeding may help normalize a very abnormal and difficult experience for the mother of a child likely to have significant long-term disabilities.

Summary

The presence of a neural tube defect does not mean an infant cannot breastfeed. If the infant is neurologically capable, it can be done. An alternative is to use expressed breastmilk.

Reference

Hurtekant KM, Spatz DL. Special considerations for breastfeeding the infant with spina bifida. J Perinat Neonatal Nurs 21:69-75, 2007.

Osteogenesis Imperfecta

This autosomal dominant condition results in extreme brittleness of the bones and occurs in about 1 in 20,000 infants. Production of abnormal type I collagen, an important component of bone, cartilage, and skin tissues is responsible for the clinical picture. Four types of osteogenesis imperfecta are recognized, with manifestations ranging from so severe that death during the neonatal period occurs to so mild that the condition is not recognized until adulthood.

Signs and Symptoms

The classic triad of manifestations for osteogenesis imperfecta are fragile bone, bluish sclerae (the whites of the eyes), and deafness. Fractures can occur *in utero*, during delivery, or may not occur until after discharge when the apparently healthy infant subsequently develops bumps, bruises, and fractures during early infancy. Child abuse may be suspected initially in a case of osteogenesis imperfecta when the infant brought for medical attention is found to have multiple unexplained fractures. Other complications associated with this condition include laxity in the joints, easy bruising, recurrent pneumonia, and cardiac failure.

Treatment

There is no curative treatment for osteogenesis imperfecta. Management focuses on trying to avoid fractures without incapacitating the individual.

Breastfeeding and Osteogenesis Imperfecta

Because of the brittleness of the bones in this condition, normal activities of holding, handling, and playing with an infant with osteogenesis imperfecta can result in bone fractures. Once recognized, a mother may become fearful of even holding her child lest she break more bones. For breastfeeding, handling and positioning the infant are important, and taking the approach of using pillows and padding to create a "platform" on which the infant can lie while the mother adjusts her position may be helpful. When the condition is so severe that family members must limit their physical interaction with the infant, breastfeeding may become the most important nurturing contact the mother has with her infant. As such, using "kangaroo care" positioning for feeding, with the infant lying prone, skin-to-skin on her chest, may be a safe way of increasing physical contact between the mother and her infant.

Summary

An infant with osteogenesis imperfecta can breastfeed, but the breastfeeding process often requires technical modification to assist the mother with safe positioning of her infant.

References

Esposito P, Plotkin II. Surgical treatment of osteogenesis imperfecta: current concepts. Curr Opin Pediatr 20:52-57, 2008.

McLean KR. Osteogenesis imperfecta. Neonatal Netw 23:7-14, 2004.

Phenylketonuria (PKU)

Phenylketonuria (PKU) is an inherited metabolic abnormality that causes an inability to metabolize the amino acid phenylalanine into the amino acid tyrosine. This results in excessive levels of phenyalanine or its abnormal metabolic products (phenylketones) in the blood, a condition that is damaging to cells in the developing central nervous system.

In the United States, the frequency of PKU is about 1:10,000. Northern European ancestry results in an increased frequency: the rate is about 1:6000 in Scotland and Ireland. Newborn screening for PKU is performed in many countries, including the US, and to be accurate, must be performed after the infant is at least 24 hours of age (i.e., adequate feeding must occur to produce elevated blood phenylalanine levels in infants with PKU).

Signs and Symptoms

In unrecognized/untreated patients, the progressive injury to the developing central nervous system by phenylalanine and phenylketones usually manifests as developmental delay in the first year of life. Ultimately, severe mental retardation occurs. In untreated patients with PKU, 95% have IQs less than 50. Other findings can include seizures, autistic behavior, eczema-like rashes, irregular skin pigmentation, shortened life span, and abnormal pigmentation. The urine and blood of patients with PKU can have a particular musty odor.

Treatment

Treatment of PKU is dietary, with the goal of minimizing the amount of ingested phenylalanine. This prevents ongoing neurologic injury and can allow normal development. Because phenylalanine is an essential amino acid (i.e., the body is unable to produce it, and some amount is required for growth and development), it cannot be totally removed from the diet. Therefore, balancing the infant's phenylalanine intake, so it is high enough for growth and development to take place, but as low as possible to minimize phenylketone production and neurologic injury, is the challenge presented, and usually requires specialized care.

Breastfeeding and PKU

Breastmilk contains less phenylalanine than infant formula, and because the infant with PKU requires some phenylalanine in their diet, it can be successfully integrated into a feeding program that combines human milk and phenylalanine-free formula. The balance between breastmilk and phenylalanine-free formula is determined by measuring the blood phenylalanine levels of the infant and changing the ratios of breastmilk to formula to keep this level in a safe range (van Rijn et al., 2003). In most cases, infants and children with PKU are followed by a physician who specializes in the care of patients with this disorder. Of note, infants who received breastmilk rather than infant formula prior to the recognition of their PKU have slightly higher IQs (about 14 points) than infants who received regular formula before their diagnosis was made (Riva et al., 1996).

While elevated blood levels of phenylalanine and phenylketones are injurious to the developing central nervous system, once the nervous system has matured, some experts suggest that liberalization of dietary phenylalanine can occur without risk, other than having elevated blood phenylalanine levels. Because elevated blood phenylalanine levels in a pregnant woman are very dangerous for the developing fetus, women of child-bearing age who were treated for PKU as children need to make this fact clear to their physicians, so that appropriate dietary measures can be instituted should they become pregnant (Purnell, 2001).

Summary

Infants with PKU can breastfeed as part of a managed program that combines human milk feeding with phenylalanine-free formula. Ongoing monitoring of the blood phenylalanine levels in infants with PKU is needed to find the correct balance between breastmilk and phenylalanine-free formula feeding.

References

Purnell H. Phenylketonuria and maternal phenylketonuria. Breastfeed Rev 9:19 21, 2001.

Riva E, Agnostoni C, Biasucci G, Trojan S, Luotti S, Fiori L, Giovannini M. Early breastfeeding is linked to higher intelligence quotient scores in dietary treated phenylketonuric children. Acta Paediatr 85:56-58, 1996.

van Rijn M, Bekhof J, Dijkstra T, Smit PG, Moddermam P, van Spronsen FJ. A different approach to breastfeeding of the infant with phenylketonuria. Eur J Pediatr 162:323-326, 2003.

Pierre Robin Sequence

The name Pierre Robin sequence refers to the triad of micrognathia (a very small jaw), glossoptosis (an irregular tongue position), and palatal abnormalities (either a high arched palate or cleft palate). The most prominent theory about the development of this pattern of abnormalities is that abnormal formation of the jaw bone predisposes to subsequent development of the tongue and palatal abnormalities in the fetus. Other congenital malformations are often seen with Pierre Robin sequence, particularly congenital glaucoma and heart anomalies. The severity of Pierre Robin sequence varies significantly from patient to patient: some patients may be so severely affected that they die in the perinatal period, while others can be managed successfully with minor interventions.

Characteristics

The very small, receding jaw bone of patients with Pierre Robin sequence results in feeding and, often, airway difficulties. Even if an adequate airway can be maintained positionally, about 40% of patients still have feeding difficulties (Smith & Senders, 2006). By age three, from 78%-92% of patients can successfully handle an oral diet (Smith & Senders, 2006). Airway difficulties are accentuated when the infant is placed on its back: the posterior rotation of the tongue causes it to fall backward and block the airway. Re-positioning maneuvers are used first to try to prevent this. Chronic airway obstruction requiring intervention beyond simple positioning maneuvers occurs in 30-60% of patients (Smith & Senders, 2006). When tracheostomy is used, dependence on this airway lasts 17-30 months, with 85% of patients successfully decanulated by age three (Smith & Senders, 2006).

Approximately 20% of patients develop mental retardation, although this may be due to early asphyxia in some instances. Chronic ear infections and gastroesophageal reflux may complicate Pierre Robin sequence and require that patients be monitored closely for middle ear disease that can lead to hearing loss and delayed speech.

Treatment

Infants with Pierre Robin sequence require careful airway and feeding management. If cleft palate is present, it requires repair. Feeding problems are common because of the anatomical abnormalities, hence, feeding by gavage tube (feeds passed into the stomach through a temporary orogastric tube) is often necessary. Use of feeding aides, such as the Haberman™ feeder, which does not require suction to deliver milk, may be beneficial. Unfortunately, the combination of feeding and airway problems may require aggressive interventions. Tracheostomy placement can relieve the chronic airway obstruction, and sometimes surgery to either attach the tongue to the lower lip, glossopexy (Denny et al., 2004), or mandibular distraction (Mandell et al., 2004) to lengthen the jaw, must be used to keep the tongue from falling back and obstructing both the esophagus and the airway. These interventions can sometimes be reversed once the child's jaw has grown enough to decrease their glossoptosis. In some instances, the infant is fed in the prone position for several months aft ⌐ birth to achieve a gravity-assisted functional reversal of glossoptosis. Such positioning obviously makes nursing very difficult.

Breastfeeding and Pierre Robin Sequence

The success of breastfeeding in this and other conditions with simultaneous airway embarrassment and oral dysfunction depends on the severity of symptoms. In most cases, successful breastfeeding is unlikely. However, feeding of expressed human milk by whatever mechanism is determined to be safest and most effective should be encouraged. Using an electric breast pump to establish and maintain the mother's milk supply should be encouraged. Despite the anatomic and functional abnormalities associated with Pierre Robin sequence, mother's milk will still provide the same benefits as provided to an infant who can breastfeed, and this may be even more important in the situation where cranio-facial abnormalities predispose to infections.

Summary

Mothers of infants with Pierre Robin sequence should be encouraged to breastfeed. If it cannot be maintained because of infant characteristics, they should be encouraged to provide expressed human milk for their infant. An electric breast pump can be used to establish lactation and maintain the mother's milk supply.

References

Denny AD, Amm CA, Schaefer RB. Outcomes of tongue-lip adhesion for neonatal respiratory distress caused by Pierre Robin sequence. J Craniofac Surg 15:819-823, 2004.

Mandell DL, Yellon RF, Bradley JP, Izadi K, Gordon CB. Mandibular distraction for micrognathia and severe upper airway obstruction. Arch Otolaryngol Head Neck Surg 130:344-348, 2004.

Smith MC, Senders CW. Prognosis of airway obstruction and feeding difficulty in Robin sequence. Int J Pediatr Otorhinolaryngol 70:319-324, 2006.

Postpartum Depression

Postpartum depression is a psychological state of a mother after delivery that meets the clinical criteria for depression. The "baby blues" is a less severe, but very common (up to 80% of new mothers) feeling of emotional distress that occurs in the first two to three days after delivery. The "baby blues" are transient, usually resolving quickly without a requirement for counseling or medications. In postpartum depression, the emotional distress is not transient, but deepens with time and requires intervention for correction.

Postpartum depression may occur in 10-20% of women. Mothers with a history of depressive illness prepartum are at higher risk of development of postpartum depression. Infrequently, depression progresses to postpartum psychosis. In postpartum depression, the mother will require emotional and psychological support. In some instances, medical treatment for the depression may be necessary, including antidepressant medication, hospitalization, and/or psychiatric counseling that are the basis for treatment of other depressive illnesses. If a breastfeeding mother develops severe postpartum depression, her illness and care can impact her ability to breastfeed because of the medications used for her treatment, potential loss of interest in her infant, and possible separation from her infant due to hospitalization. Needless to say, every effort should be made to allow breastfeeding to continue through this time.

Causes

The reason new mothers experience the "baby blues" immediately postpartum is not completely understood. The hormonal changes that occur with the cessation of pregnancy, the emotional highs and lows associated with the major life change of having a baby, or the uncovering of deeper underlying social/emotional issues by the birth of a child may all contribute to the process. Specific situations, such as a negative or disappointing birth experience, a fussy and/or demanding infant, difficulties establishing nursing, or inadequate social support systems for the new mother or alienation from existing support systems have all been associated with developing the "blues." The "blues" usually last only a few days after delivery, but may persist for a week or two at the outside.

Postpartum depression is a clinical condition that develops insidiously over the first several weeks postpartum until it is recognized, usually two to six weeks after delivery. Mothers who suffer from postpartum depression begin with the "baby blues," but their feelings become persistent and debilitating to the point of clinical depression. The risk factors for development of postpartum depression include a previous history of depression or postpartum depression, a family history of depression, difficulties adjusting to motherhood, single parent status, problems with infant bonding soon after delivery, and feelings of loss of control. Determination of whether any of these factors are present should be done both pre- and in the immediate postpartum period, as their recognition facilitates early intervention if depression develops.

Postpartum psychosis is more rare (1-2/1000 mothers) and is the most severe postpartum psychological disorder. It can have a dramatic onset within two to three days of delivery, but in most women its symptoms appear over the first two weeks following delivery. It presents as a complete departure from reality by the mother. It may require hospitalization, medication, and/or regular psychiatric care.

Signs and Symptoms

Mothers with the "baby blues" feel overwhelmed and fatigued. They are sometimes tearful and often lack confidence in their mothering skills. They may feel sad, suffer from insomnia, be anxious, have reduced appetite, or have feelings of ambivalence for their infant in the first several days after delivery. These feelings do not interfere with the mother's ability to function or care for her infant. The usual course of this process is for the mother to gradually regain control and confidence in herself and learn to manage the new responsibilities of motherhood.

The manifestations of postpartum depression include sadness, loss of pleasure, mood swings, lack of attachment to the baby, general lack of interest in life, panic, fatigue, persistent crying, sleep pattern changes, and hopelessness. The depression generally becomes recognizable about two to four weeks postpartum, but can also develop later. The duration of the clinical depression is variable: resolution over about two weeks has been described, but most cases persist for longer periods of time.

Postpartum psychosis presents as irrational ideas or thoughts, feelings of failure, thoughts of suicide, hallucinations, violent behavior, threats of harm to self or the new baby, lack of control, and separation from reality. Because of the severity of this illness, it is imperative that this mother be identified and treated immediately.

Management/Treatment

Mothers who suffer from mild disorders, such as the "baby blues," often only need social support and reassurance from their families and friends. They need to be told that they are exhibiting good mothering skills, and emphasis should be placed on what they are doing right. Social support systems (home visitations, peer support) and resources to assist the mother in managing her other responsibilities, such as household chores and cooking, help alleviate feelings of being overwhelmed and allow the mother to focus on herself and her new baby. Instructing the mother on appropriate coping mechanisms for her social or home environment can help her to resume the regular activities of daily life. These mothers should be encouraged to continue breastfeeding, with support from a lactation consultant if feeding difficulties occur.

Management of mothers with postpartum depression is highly dependent on the severity of the illness. Options range from concentrated emotional support for mothers with mild depression to use of antidepressant medications and treatments for those more severely affected. Social support is usually a component of treatment, and recent evidence suggests exercise and inclusion of omega-3 fatty acids in the diet may be beneficial for treatment of depression (Shaw & Kaczorowski, 2007). Psychosocial and psychological counseling (Dennis & Hodnett, 2007) and antidepressant medication are effective and often part of the treatment. Mothers need to be re-evaluated on a regular basis for signs of response to treatment, and their infants need to be assessed regularly for adequacy of feeding and appropriate growth and weight gain (Rahman et al., 2004).

Mothers who develop postpartum psychosis need immediate medical attention, as they may be at risk for harming themselves or their babies. This diagnosis requires pharmacologic therapy, psychiatric counseling, and possibly hospitalization as a part of treatment. This condition obviously stresses the mother-infant relationship in many ways, including continuation of breastfeeding. If separated from her infant, a mother with this condition should be given the opportunity to maintain her milk supply through a pumping regimen. However, the priority is to ensure the safety of both mother and baby.

Because motherhood is expected to be filled with happiness, some new mothers feel ashamed or uneasy revealing that they are having problems with unhappy thoughts and feelings. As a result, the signs may be subtle because they are actively being hidden. Being open with the mother in this situation, expressing concern for her and her infant's well-being, and emphasizing that postpartum mood disorders are not voluntary on the part of the mother may help get the mother to seek medical assistance.

Breastfeeding and Postpartum Depression

Mood disorders in the postpartum period range from the "baby blues" to severe postpartum psychosis. Periods of tearfulness or feelings of being overwhelmed are normal in the first few days after delivery. These should fade as the mother becomes confident in her mothering skills and learns to manage the new challenges in her life. However, some mothers progress and develop postpartum depression. This depression, depending on its severity, can be managed through counseling, developing coping strategies, diet and lifestyle changes, or antidepressant medication use. Further deterioration of postpartum depression to postpartum psychosis raises concerns for injury to the mother and/or her baby, and thus may also require hospitalization. If a mother requires antidepressant medications, there are several on the market that are compatible with breastfeeding. In all cases, mothers should be encouraged and supported in their efforts to breastfeed, and efforts should be made to allow breastfeeding to continue if acceptable to the mother.

Summary

Mothers with postpartum depression can continue to breastfeed. Mild cases of the baby blues usually fade as the mother becomes more confident in her parenting abilities. More severe forms of depression require some form of intervention, such as counseling, coping strategies, diet and lifestyle changes, antidepressants, and on occasion, hospitalization when necessary. Mothers with postpartum depression who wish to continue breastfeeding require emotional support and encouragement for their efforts.

References

Dennis CL, Hodnett E. Psychosocial and psychological interventions for treating postpartum depression. Cochrane Database Syst Rev Oct 17: CD006116, 2007.

Rahman A, Iqbal Z, Bunn J, Lovel H, Harrington R. Impact of maternal depression on infant nutritional status and illness: a cohort study. Arch Gen Psychiatry 61:946-952, 2004.

Shaw E, Kaczorowski J. Postpartum care - what's new? Curr Opin Obstet Gynecol 19:561-567, 2007.

Primary Dysmenorrhea (Menstrual Cramps)

Primary dysmenorrhea, or menstrual cramps, is a common problem; however, its true incidence is difficult to determine because definitions vary. Current estimates of its prevalence vary from 45-95% of all women. It appears to be the most common gynecological problem, regardless of age or nationality (Proctor & Farquhar, 2006). It occurs just before and/or during the first several days of the menstrual cycle and is due to excessive or imbalanced uterine prostaglandin production, which stimulates both uterine contractions and local ischemia. It is differentiated from "secondary" dysmenorrhea in that "primary" dysmenorrhea has no evident cause to explain it, while "secondary" dysmenorrhea is associated with either anatomical abnormalities or with diseases of the pelvic organs.

Causes

While in the past primary dysmenorrhea was ascribed to either psychological or emotional causes, more recent information indicates it is likely due to uterine production of prostaglandins. When the tissue lining the uterus is lost as menstruation begins, this tissue releases prostaglandins. Women with the most severe dysmenorrhea have higher levels of prostaglandins in their menstrual fluid. The effect of these prostaglandins is to stimulate frequent, often dysrhythmic contraction of the uterine muscles, producing the cramping pain (Dawood, 2006). A number of factors are associated with its occurrence: these include age less than 30 years, low body mass index, smoking, menarche before twelve years old, longer menstrual cycles, heavier menstrual flow, never having had a child, premenstrual syndrome, sterilization, and pelvic inflammatory disease. Factors that appear to be protective against it are younger age at first childbirth, oral contraceptive use, and regular exercise (Latthe et al., 2006). The syndrome is often under-diagnosed and under-treated because many women self-treat their symptoms without seeking medical assistance.

Signs and Symptoms

Women report severe lower abdominal cramping with sharp, intermittent spasms of pain. Some women may experience pain that radiates to the lower back and/or the thighs. Other symptoms may include nausea and vomiting, fatigue, diarrhea, and/or headache. Primary dysmenorrhea is not the same as "premenstrual syndrome." The former produces symptoms at the onset of menstruation while the latter, which includes breast tenderness, pain, and abdominal bloating, occurs prior to the start of the cycle and relents as menstrual flow begins.

Management/Treatment

Women who present with severe dysmenorrhea should have a medical evaluation to rule out "secondary" dysmenorrhea due to an anatomical abnormality of a pelvic disease process (such as endometriosis or pelvic inflammatory disease). Nonsteroidal anti-inflammatory drugs (NSAIDs) directly block synthesis of prostaglandins, and are, therefore, excellent drugs for treatment of primary dysmenorrhea. Acetaminophen also has a beneficial effect, but it is not as strong as the effects of NSAID medications. Ibuprofen is the NSAID of choice for nursing mothers. If NSAID medications are not effective, some physicians will prescribe oral contraceptive medications to control the menstrual cycle (and hence the production of uterine prostaglandin). Because the use of oral contraceptive medications containing estrogen may negatively impact the milk supply, use of NSAIDS by breastfeeding mothers to control their dysmenorrhea is preferred. If a mother does not get adequate pain relief using NSAID medications alone, addition of alternative approaches to pain relief, such as acupuncture or transcutaneous electrical nerve stimulation, may be beneficial (Proctor et al., 2002). Topical application of a heating pad to the lower abdomen, in association with NSAIDS use, can also provide relief (Akin et al., 2001).

Breastfeeding and Primary Dysmenorrhea

Breastfeeding may continue when women suffer from severe cramping. Care should be taken to ensure that medications used for its treatment are compatible with breastfeeding. Primary dysmenorrhea is not a contraindication for breastfeeding.

Summary

Primary dysmenorrhea is estimated to affect approximately 90% of women. It can be very painful for women, but many times responds positively to the use of NSAIDs. Breastfeeding mothers should continue to nurse their baby and use ibuprofen as the preferred method of pain relief. Any other medications should be evaluated by the mother's physician for compatibility with breastfeeding.

References

Akin MD, Weingand KW, Hengehold DA, Goodale MB, Hinkle RT, Smith RP. Continuous low-level topical heat in the treatment of dysmenorrhea. Obstet Gynecol 97:343-349, 2001.

Dawood MY. Primary dysmenorrhea: advances in pathogenesis and management. Obstet Gynecol 108:428-441, 2006.

Latthe P, Mihnini L, Gray R, Hills R, Khan K. Factors predisposing women to chronic pelvic pain: systematic review. BMJ 332:749-55, 2006. Epub 2006 Feb 16.

Proctor M, Farquhar C. Diagnosis and management of dysmenorrhea. Br Med J 332:11344-11348, 2006.

Proctor ML, Smith CA, Farquhar CM, Stones RW. Transcutaneous electrical nerve stimulation and acupuncture for primary dysmenorrhea. Cochrane Database Syst. Rev. CD002123, 2002.

Psoriasis

Psoriasis is a chronic skin condition with a pattern of exacerbation and remission that results from abnormally rapid turnover of the epidermis. Its specific cause is unknown. It occurs in 1-3% of the US population. Approximately 10% of cases appear in early childhood (before age ten), and 35% of cases appear before age 20. Physical trauma to the skin, sunburn, stress, infections, and certain medications (e.g., beta-blockers, lithium) trigger or worsen psoriatic skin changes.

Signs and Symptoms

The usual skin lesions of psoriasis are red and scaly, and typically occur on the scalp, chest, knees, elbows, extensor surfaces of the limbs, buttocks, low back, and on the genitalia. The lesions start as small erythematous papules with a fine scaly surface. As the lesions progress, well demarcated plaques form that vary in size and severity. There is a tendency for the plaques to occur symmetrically on the body. The plaques are described as "silvery" and often their edges lift free of the skin surface. If a plaque is removed, a punctate bleeding site (Auspitz's sign) appears where the plaque had been attached. Pitting of the nails occurs in up to 50% of patients, and arthritis is seen in 5-10% of cases. Psoriatic involvement of the nipple/breast is described.

Treatment

No curative treatment for psoriasis is known. The types, locations, and extent of lesions influence the type of treatment used. Exposure to sunlight has a striking beneficial effect on psoriasis, and patients often spontaneously improve in the summer. Use of ultraviolet B irradiation alone or in combination with coal tar or anthralin may be used. Topical treatment with coal tar, vitamin D analogs, and retinoids are all used. In severe cases, systemic retinoids and methotrexate are sometimes used.

Breastfeeding and Psoriasis Medications

Psoriasis is not transmitted by contact. The topical medications usually prescribed have little systemic absorption, but it may be prudent to avoid widespread intensive use during breastfeeding and to avoid direct applications to the nipples to minimize exposure of the infant's skin to these medications. If topical medications must be used on the nipple, temporary cessation of breastfeeding from the affected breast may be necessary, with the baby continuing to nurse from the unaffected side. The mother can maintain milk production on the affected side by pumping. If topical retinoids are needed, tazarotene may be preferable to etretinate because unlike etretinate, tazarotene is poorly absorbed through the skin and, therefore, unlikely to affect a breastfeeding infant.

Breastfeeding and Psoriasis

Some of the medications used to treat psoriasis, rather than the condition itself, can be problematic for breastfeeding women. The use of anti-psoriasis medications and breastfeeding should be discussed with the mother's dermatologist.

Summary

For the mother with psoriasis, breastfeeding is appropriate as long as the medications being used for treatment are safe for the nursing infant.

Reference

Rollman O, Pihl-Lundin I. Acitretin excretion into breast milk. Acta Derm Venereol 70:487-490, 1990.

Pyloric Stenosis

In some infants, hypertrophy (thickening) of the muscular wall surrounding the portion of the stomach that enters the small intestine (the pylorus) can narrow the passage way and block passage of food and fluid out of the stomach. This condition is called "pyloric stenosis." It is the most common condition requiring surgery in the first months of life. There is often a family history of the problem, and the preponderance of cases occurs in first born male infants. Recent epidemiologic studies suggest that use of the antibiotic erythromycin (which has significant effects on stimulating gastric contraction) in infants in the first two weeks of life increases the relative risk of developing pyloric stenosis approximately ten-fold (Mahon et al., 2001). Whether erythromycin use by lactating women has an association remains unclear.

Signs and Symptoms

Persistent, non-bilious, projectile vomiting within the first three months of life is the most common presentation for this condition. The parents' descriptions often emphasize the forcefulness of the vomiting - "...it shot across the room" - which clearly differentiates it from chalasia, the "spitting" type of regurgitation that nearly all infants have. Initially, despite the episode of vomiting, the infant eagerly goes back to feeding, but with repeated episodes, they can become irritable and weak. Continued vomiting leads to decreased urine output, and eventually weight loss, dehydration, and sometimes electrolyte imbalances (hypochloremic alkalosis) can occur. The picture is different from the infant with vomiting due to overfeeding, who continues to feed and thrive despite the vomiting.

In some infants, experts are able to feel a hypertrophied pyloric muscle when the abdomen is examined. This is commonly referred to as "feeling the olive" because the hypertrophied muscle is approximately that size. When examined by sonography, the hypertrophied pyloric muscle can be demonstrated in about 90% of cases.

Treatment

A pyloromyotomy is performed to correct the pyloric stenosis. In this procedure, the surgeon cuts through the pyloric muscle (without entering the bowel lumen) on one side, which immediately removes the obstruction to stomach emptying. Because some children are dehydrated and in electrolyte imbalance at the time their diagnosis is made, intravenous fluid treatment is often given for 24 hours before this corrective surgery is performed to ensure the infant is optimally prepared to undergo surgery.

Breastfeeding and Pyloric Stenosis

Breastfeeding has no clear impact *per se* on the development or prevention of pyloric stenosis. Usually, recovery after pyloromyotomy is prompt, and there is essentially no or minimal interruption to breastfeeding. Postoperatively allowing *ad libitum* feeds rather than having a gradually increasing feeding program decreases the time to full diet and discharge (Garza et al., 2002). As with other conditions where breastfeeding may be transiently interrupted, the mother can maintain her milk supply by pumping, and the pumped milk stored to be given to the infant once feeding is re-established.

References

Garza JJ, Morash D, Dzakovic A, Mondschein JK, Jaksic T. Ad libitum feeding decreases hospital stay for neonates after pyloromyotomy. J Pediatr Surg 37:493-495, 2002.

Mahon BE, Rosenman MB, Kleiman MB. Maternal and infant use of erythromycin and other macrolide antibiotics as risk factors for infantile hypertrophic pyloric stenosis. J Pediatr 139:380-384, 2001.

Rabies

Rabies is an animal-borne infection that is usually transmitted to humans through injury (bites, scratches) inflicted by an infected animal. The animal's saliva is the source of the virus. Many types of animals can be infected with rabies virus, but several types are notorious for this. Depending on the geographic location, skunks, foxes, raccoons, coyotes, cats (currently the most commonly identified rabid animal), or dogs may be the primary reservoir. All bats are considered infected with rabies. In some areas, rabies is common in domesticated livestock. Local health departments are the best sources for regional information on animal carriage of rabies and management of animal exposures. It is important to realize that an animal need not appear ill to be able to transmit rabies. Transmission to humans from small rodents and lagomorphs (rabbits) is rare. The incubation period between exposure to development of clinical symptoms can vary from days to years (depending on how far the virus must travel from the inoculation site to reach the central nervous system), with the result that the exposure episode for some cases of rabies may have occurred months to a year before illness and may never be clearly identified.

Signs and Symptoms

Rabies virus infection causes brain inflammation (encephalitis). Initial signs are non-specific: headache, fever, malaise. Vomiting may occur, and before onset of encephalitis, the patient may complain of pain or paresthesia (numbness) at the site of the animal bite. The disease then progresses to include changes in personality and behavior: agitation, hyperactivity, anxiety, and sometimes hydrophobia (fear of drinking water because rabies-induced swallowing muscle incoordination results in choking). In many patients, "lucid episodes" occur between periods of altered behavior and personality. Dysphagia and hypersalivation because of swallowing muscle incoordination, occur in about 50% of cases. The disease then progresses to stupor, coma, and death due to progressive brain infection and encephalitis.

Treatment

One case of (relatively) successful treatment/survival of clinical rabies using a medically induced coma has been reported (Willoughby et al., 2005). In general, prevention/avoidance is a much more effective approach to this condition than treatment. In the instance where a high risk bite occurs, initial treatment should include cleaning the wound with soap and water. Capture the animal if possible, either observe it for development of rabies if time allows, or destroy it and examine its brain for rabies infection. Depending on the situation and the advice of the physician, the bitten individual should either await results of animal testing or immediately start rabies post-exposure prophylaxis treatment. This includes two components: injections of human rabies immunoglobulin (half the dose infiltrated at the wound site, the other half given intramuscularly), and initiation of the five dose rabies vaccination series (intramuscular injections on days 0, 3, 7, 14, and 28). If examination of the animal brain is negative, the immunization series need not be completed.

Veterinarians and others individuals who are routinely exposed to wild animals should receive pre-exposure prophylaxis (three dose rabies vaccination series) against rabies.

Breastfeeding and Rabies

Human-to-human transmission of rabies has only been documented to occur through cornea transplantation. If a breastfeeding mother is exposed to rabies, she should immediately initiate appropriate post-exposure prophylaxis, and breastfeeding can resume/continue once this has started. There are no concerns regarding rabies vaccine exposure to the nursing infant.

Summary

If a breastfeeding mother is exposed to rabies, she can continue to breastfeed once the appropriate post-exposure prophylaxis has been initiated.

Reference

Willoughby RE Jr, Tieves KS, Hoffman GM, et al. Survival after treatment for rabies with induction of coma. N Engl J Med 352:2508-2514, 2005.

Rickets

Rickets is a disease that results from lack of vitamin D. Vitamin D is important for bone matrix mineralization and is characterized by inadequate bone matrix mineralization.

Between birth and six months of age, the infant receives vitamin D from their diet, synthesizes vitamin D from sunlight exposure, and utilizes stores of vitamin D transferred transplacentally to the fetus. If inadequate exposure to sunlight is a concern, some experts recommend a daily vitamin D intake of 200-400 IU (American Academy of Pediatrics, 2005).

Vitamin D is needed for maintenance of a healthy skeleton throughout life. Its major function is to maintain the extracellular concentrations of calcium and phosphorus in their normal ranges. To do this, vitamin D enhances the efficiency of absorption of dietary calcium and phosphorus from the small intestine. If dietary intake of calcium and phosphorus are inadequate to maintain their normal extracellular concentrations, vitamin D and parathyroid hormone act together to mobilize calcium and phosphate from stores in the bone.

Vitamin D comes either from the diet or is synthesized in the skin via sunlight exposure. Relatively few foods are naturally rich in vitamin D: fish liver oils, the flesh of fatty fish, and the liver and fat of aquatic mammals (e.g., seals and polar bears). Because none of these foods is prominent in the typical western diet, fortification of foods with vitamin D, in particular cow's milk, is routine in the developed world. In addition, some cereals, breads, and margarines are also vitamin D fortified. Cow's milk-based infant formulas are fortified with vitamin D by law (400 IU/L). In contrast, breastmilk contains 22-40 IU/L.

A recent summary of nutritional rickets in US children less than 18 years old between 1986-2003 (Weisberg et al., 2004) noted that in 166 cases, 96% were breastfed infants, 83% were described as black or African American, and only 5% of the breastfed infants were receiving vitamin D supplementation. This study had a large impact on new recommendations for vitamin D supplementation of breastfed infants as described below.

Signs and Symptoms

The clinical manifestations of rickets are progressive deformities of the skeleton, enlargement of the wrists and ankles, enlargement of the joints of the long bones and rib cage, head enlargement, curvature of the thighs and spine, generalized muscle weakness, short stature, and hypocalcemic seizures. Other classical findings in rickets include "craniotabes" (a skull that is so thinned that pressure on it causes indentation that springs back when pressure is relieved, similar to what occurs with a ping-pong ball), "rachitic rosary" (obvious enlargement of the joints between the ribs and the costochondral cartilages), "caput quadratum" (a box-like shaping of the head due to flattening of the skull caused by pressure when lying down), "pigeon breast" (forward projection of the sternum), "knock-knees" deformities, and leg bowing.

Diagnosis

Radiographic examination of the wrist is useful for early diagnosis of rickets because the changes in the radius and ulna often appear early in the course of the disease. In rickets, the distal ends of these bones become cupped, widened, and frayed and the density of the bone shaft decreases. Prior to development of bone changes, biochemical changes are present in the blood. These include decreased serum calcium levels, elevated parathyroid hormone levels, and elevated alkaline phosphatase levels, while the serum phosporus levels remain normal. With progression of disease, serum phosphorus levels may drop and calcium levels may normalize. In the most severe cases, serum calcium and phosphorus are low, alkaline phosphatase and parathyroid hormone levels are elevated, and vitamin D levels are low.

Treatment

The skeletal effects of rickets can be reversed by treatment with vitamin D. The dose used depends on the severity of the rickets. Prevention of rickets requires adequate amounts of dietary vitamin D supplementation or enough sunlight exposure to allow synthesis of needed vitamin D. Vitamin D supplementation to infants in the US is usually provided in combination with vitamins A and C.

Breastfeeding and Rickets

The American Academy of Pediatrics recommends that all breastfed infants receive daily vitamin D supplementation of 200 IU beginning during the first two months of life, and this should be continued until consumption of vitamin D fortified formula or milk is at least 500 mL/day.

Summary

Rickets is caused by a lack of vitamin D. All breastfed infants should receive 200 IU vitamin D as a daily supplement, beginning in the first two months of life, and this should continue until their intake of vitamin D supplemented milk is adequate to replace the daily vitamin D dose.

References

American Academy of Pediatrics Section on Breastfeeding. Breastfeeding and the use of human milk. Pediatrics 115:496-506, 2005.

Weisberg P, Scanlon KS, Li R, Cogswell ME. Nutritional rickets among children in the United States: review of cases reported between 1986 and 2003. Am J Clin Nutr 80(6 suppl): 1697S-1705S, 2004.

Rubella

German measles, the common name for rubella, is a mild childhood illness that is now rare because of immunization. In the past, infection usually occurred in childhood with resultant life-long immunity, and for children, it was a nuisance illness rather than a threatening one. However, if infection failed to occur in childhood and instead occurred early in pregnancy, congenital rubella, with its associated cardiac malformations, deafness, eye malformations, and neurological injury, occurred in up to 50% of infants. The severity and frequency of congenital rubella syndrome is the greatest threat caused by this disease.

Signs and Symptoms

Illness in children and adults is associated with rash, low grade fever, and lymphadenopathy that usually resolves in three to five days. Enlargement of the suboccipital, posterior auricular, and cervical nodes is common. The virus typically replicates in the nasopharynx, so that respiratory droplet secretions are the likely mechanism for transmission. Individuals with rubella are most infectious several days before the onset of rash.

When infection occurs in a pregnant woman, the most common congenital anomalies in the infant are ophthalmologic (cataracts, microphthalmia, glaucoma, retinopathy), cardiac (patent ductus arteriosus and pulmonary stenosis), auditory (sensorineural deafness), and neurologic (American Academy of Pediatrics, 2006). Other findings suggestive of congenital infections in general, "blueberry muffin" skin lesions, hepatosplenomegaly, and jaundice, can also occur. Infants born with congenital rubella can be infectious for a year or more, and precautions should be taken to prevent exposure of pregnant women to them.

Treatment

No specific treatment is available for rubella. Immunization against rubella in childhood is now routine. Rubella vaccine is a component in the MMR immunization.

Breastfeeding and Rubella

Rubella virus has been isolated from breastmilk during maternal rubella infection and following rubella immunization of lactating women. Antibodies against rubella are also found in milk. When infants who were either breastfed or bottle-fed after their mothers received rubella vaccine were tested, 56% of the breastfed, and 0% of the bottle-fed infants had either infectious virus or virus antigen recovered from them, indicating a strong association with breastfeeding. Twenty-five percent of the breastfed infants and 0% of the bottle-fed infants also showed transient seroconversion to rubella virus (Losonsky et al., 1982). However, it is unclear from these studies whether transmission of the rubella vaccine virus to the infant occurred via breast or whether acquisition from the vaccinated mother occurred via another (e.g., respiratory droplet) route. According to current recommendations from the Centers for Disease Control and Prevention "Neither inactivated nor live vaccines administered to a lactating woman affect the safety of breastfeeding for mothers or infants" (Atkinson et al., 2002).

Summary
The mother who has rubella or who has received rubella vaccine can continue to breastfeed.

References

American Academy of Pediatrics. Rubella. In: Pickering LK, Baker CJ, Long SS, McMillan JA, eds. Redbook: 2006 Report of the Committee on Infectious Diseases. 27th edition. Elk Grove Village, IL: American Academy of Pediatrics, 2006: pp 574-579.

Atkinson WL, Pickering LK, Schwartz B, Weniger BG, Iskander JK, Watson JC. General recommendations on immunization. MMWR 51(RR02):1-36, 2002.

Losonsky GA, Fishaut JM, Strussenberg J, Ogra PL. Effect of immunization against rubella on lactation products. II. Maternal-neonatal interactions. J Infect Dis 145:661-666, 1982.

Salmonellosis

While gastroenteritis in infants and small children can result from a large variety of infectious agents, most are viruses that cause illnesses whose major threat to health is development of dehydration. Less frequently, gastroenteritis in infants is caused by bacterial pathogens, such as *Salmonella*, *Shigella*, or *Campylobacter*, which cause dysenteric (bloody diarrhea), gastrointestinal disorders, and occasionally, invasive infections. Infection caused by *Salmonella* is of particular significance because of its tendency to cause invasive disease (particularly meningitis) in infants less than three months old.

Salmonella organisms are spread by fecal-oral contamination. Reptiles and birds are well known reservoirs of *Salmonella* in nature, but many types of animals carry them. Transmission to humans after contact with animals is common, emphasizing the importance of hand washing following interaction or contact with animals.

Signs and Symptoms

In general, two forms of Salmonellosis are recognized: gastroenteritis and enteric fever. In the former, acute onset with fever and gastrointestinal symptoms (nausea, dysenteric diarrhea, cramps) predominate, at times accompanied by blood stream invasion. In the latter, more gradual onset of fever with headache, nausea, malaise, lethargy, diarrhea (in children), and abdominal pain occur, and blood stream invasion is the rule. Typhoid fever caused by *Salmonella typhi* is the best known enteric fever syndrome. Development of distant infection in bone, joints, or meningitis can occur in either form.

Diagnosis

Culture of *Salmonella* from the stool, blood, or bone marrow establishes the diagnosis.

Treatment

Antibiotic treatment of adults and older children with uncomplicated *Salmonella* gastroenteritis (i.e., no blood stream invasion) is not recommended because while it resolves gastroenteritis more quickly, it also causes prolonged fecal carriage and shedding of the *Salmonella*. In infants less than three months old, antibiotic treatment is usually recommended even for uncomplicated gastroenteritis because of the increased risk of developing invasive disease in this age group. Invasive *Salmonella* disease always requires antibiotic treatment (usually intravenously administered for infants) and careful observation for development of distant sites of infection.

Breastfeeding and Salmonellosis

Women with salmonellosis can breastfeed with the knowledge that there is some risk of transmission to the nursing infant because of the intimacy of breastfeeding. In addition, *Salmonella* has been isolated from breastmilk that transmitted infection (Qutaishat et al., 2003) and from milk fed to an infant who developed *Salmonella* meningitis (Chen et al., 2005), indicating transmission of *Salmonella* strains via breastmilk can occur. If a lactating mother develops uncomplicated salmonellosis, antibiotic treatment is not indicated, but careful attention to both hand washing and personal hygiene are appropriate, as is observation of the infant for any signs of infection.

Breastfeeding decreases the risk of salmonellosis in infants (Rowe et al., 2004).

Summary

Women with salmonellosis can breastfeed. Antibiotic treatment is not indicated for uncomplicated *Salmonella* gastroenteritis, but is frequently given to infants less than three months of age because of the increased risk of developing invasive *Salmonella* infection. Good hand washing and personal hygiene are important for preventing mother-to-infant transmission.

References

Chen TL, Thien PF, Liaw SC, Fung CP, Siu LK. First report of Salmonella enterica serotype panama meningitis associated with consumption of contaminated breast milk by a neonate. J Clin Microbiol 43:5400-5402, 2005.

Qutaishat SS, Stemper ME, Spencer SK, Borchardt MA, Opitz JC, Monson TA, Anderson JL, Ellingson JL. Transmission of Salmonella enterica serotype typhimurium DT104 to infants through mother's milk. Pediatrics 111:1442-1446, 2003.

Rowe SY, Rocourt JR, Shiferaw B, Kassenborg HD, Segler SD, Marcus R, Daily PJ, Hardnett FP, Slutsker L, Emerging Infections Program FeedNet Working Group. Breast-feeding decreases the risk of sporadic salmonellosis among infants in FoodNet sites. Clin Infect Dis 38(suppl3):S262-S270, 2004.

Sheehan's Syndrome

The occurrence of obstetric hemorrhage with vascular collapse followed by pituitary infarction and panhypopituitarism is called Sheehan's syndrome. Ischemia of the pituitary gland due to the hemorrhage is thought to underlie the subsequent evolution of pituitary injury and hypofunction. The lateral aspects of the pituitary gland, where most lactotrophs (prolactin-producing cells) are found, have a tenuous blood supply. Hypertrophy of these cells during pregnancy, in preparation for lactation, makes them more sensitive to ischemia. Ischemia-induced necrosis of the pituitary stalk usually stops prolactin production which leads to lactation failure. Depending on the amount of injury sustained, hypopituitarism may be immediate, may be delayed in onset for years, or may spontaneously reverse.

Signs and Symptoms

The degree of pituitary injury likely influences the timing and severity of clinical manifestations (Barkan, 1989). Following severe injury, the earliest signs of Sheehan's syndrome are usually lactation failure due to prolactin deficiency with failure to resume menses due to hypogonadism (Sert et al., 2003). Sparse regrowth of shaved pubic hair is seen for the same reason. However, with lesser injury, lactation may be successful and development of signs of pituitary insufficiency may be so subtle they take years to be appreciated. Secondary hypothyroidism, secondary adrenal failure, hypogonadotrophic hypogonadism, and growth hormone deficiency are all common in Sheehan syndrome (Sert et al., 2003), but their onset and/or recognition may be delayed as long as thirty years. Central diabetes insipidus also occurs, but is infrequent.

Treatment

Because hypopituitarism resulting from Sheehan's Syndrome can vary in severity and degree of endocrinologic abnormalities, proper management usually requires delineation of the extent of endocrine dysfunction and appropriate replacement of the deficient hormones. Evaluation of a patient with Sheehan's Syndrome is best performed by an endocrinologist who can determine the types and quantities of replacement hormones needed.

Breastfeeding and Sheehan's Syndrome

Because the hormones prolactin and oxytocin are produced by the pituitary gland, and these hormones are crucial for successful lactation, injury to the pituitary gland as occurs in Sheehan's syndrome commonly results in lactational failure. Prolactin acts on the breast to stimulate milk production, and oxytocin mediates the milk ejection reflex (milk let down) that is required for effective release of milk from the breast. The first endocrine disorder recognized to cause lactation failure is Sheehan's syndrome. If a mother has a history of peripartum hemorrhage and fails to produce enough milk or if an infant is latching on well to the breast, nursing frequently, but is failing to gain weight, Sheehan's syndrome should be a consideration. Because of the multiple trophic effects of pituitary hormones for stable physiology and survival and due to the availability of replacement hormones, the earlier Sheehan's syndrome is diagnosed, the lower the ultimate morbidity for the mother.

Summary

Sheehan's syndrome can cause lactation failure.

References

Barkan AL. Pituitary atrophy in patients with Sheehan's syndrome. Am J Med 298: 38-40, 1989.

Sert M, Tetiker T, Kirim S, Kocak M. Clinical report of 28 patients with Sheehan's syndrome. Endocrine J 50:297-301, 2003.

Sickle Cell Disease

Sickle cell disease is an inherited disorder in which an abnormal form of hemoglobin, the protein in red blood cells that carries oxygen, causes these cells to take on a sickle shape. This shape results in a diminished ability of the red blood cells to pass through the smallest blood vessels; instead, they block these blood vessels leading to poor oxygenation of the tissues. The results are "pain crises," loss of splenic function, ischemic injury to tissues, such as lung and brain, and a shortened survival. The disease occurs in many population groups, but is most common in blacks of African descent. About 8% of Black Americans are carriers for sickle cell disease, i.e., they have sickle cell "trait," which is usually an asymptomatic condition.

Signs and Symptoms

Adults and children with sickle cell disease suffer from chronic hemolytic anemia (hemoglobin levels in the 5-9 g/dL range). Spontaneous sickling of the red blood cells can cause diminished flow by vascular obstruction, which causes tissue hypoxia and pain. If these effects persist, fever, dehydration, and acidosis result, which further accentuates the red blood cells' tendencies to sickle. This self-propagating pathology results in development of "crisis," which are classified as either vaso-occlusive, sequestration, pain, or aplastic. In vaso-occlusive crisis, blood vessel obstruction results in ischemia, hypoxic injury, and tissue necrosis. In sequestration crisis, large amounts of sickled cells and blood pool in the abdominal organs, particularly the spleen, causing rapidly progressive anemia. In aplastic crisis, viral infection (usually parvovirus B19) of the bone marrow causes failure of production of red blood cells. In pain crisis, severe pain results from vascular occlusion and tissue ischemia, without obvious infarctive effects.

The ongoing vascular obstruction and tissue injury of sickle cell disease results in several clinical manifestations across time. Dactylitis, infarctive changes in the small bones of the hands and feet, manifested by symmetric pain and swelling, usually occurs in toddlers. Frontal bossing - enlargement of the boney forehead due to increased blood cell production in that area of the skull bone - becomes obvious in early childhood. Splenic function is usually lost by three to four years of age via "auto-splenectomy," due to infarctive changes in this organ. Because splenic function disappears early, individuals with sickle cell disease are particularly prone to infection caused by organisms that the spleen normally filters out of the blood and destroys - most notably *Streptococcus pneumoniae*. In addition, they have a predilection toward osteomyelitis and joint infections caused by *Salmonella* species.

Treatment

The repetitive episodes of vaso-occlusive and pain crises frequently require hospitalization for pain control, hydration, oxygenation, and antibiotic administration. Children with sickle cell disease are treated prophylactically with penicillin (to prevent *S. pneumoniae* infection) and folic acid (to ensure hematopoiesis can continue). They should also be fully immunized. No treatment except bone marrow transplantation is curative. Chronic transfusion therapy and treatment with hydroxyurea are used in some patients to try to decrease ongoing tissue injury.

Breastfeeding and Sickle Cell Disease

Breastfeeding is appropriate for the infant with sickle cell disease because of its anti-infective characteristics. It is unproven whether breastfeeding infants with sickle cell disease longer than recommended has any additional benefit.

The woman with sickle cell disease who wants to breastfeed should be supported in her decision. She should be advised to pay particular attention to her hydration state during lactation, particularly when she herself suffers from a crisis. Pain medications used to treat the crisis, including acetaminophen, codeine, and others used in these situations, are usually compatible with breastfeeding.

Summary

Women and infants with Sickle Cell Disease can breastfeed.

Syphilis

Syphilis is a sexually transmitted disease that, if untreated, results in life-long and progressively more injurious infection. The causative agent, *Treponema pallidum*, cannot be grown by routine culture methods, resulting in detection and monitoring of disease by measurement of antibody levels. Acquiring syphilis does not result in development of immunity: *T. pallidum* infection can be acquired repeatedly, and the risks are the same with each acquisition.

Signs and Symptoms

Syphilis is divided into three stages: primary, secondary, and tertiary. The primary stage is when the infection is acquired: a moist, painless ulcer at the site of entry called a chancre is the clinical characteristic of this stage. Chancres can occur on any part of the body. In women, a chancre can go unnoticed when it is located within the vagina or on the cervix. The chancre usually heals over in 14-21 days and the patient is asymptomatic. During this time, the *T. pallidum* begins to spread throughout the body. Weeks to months after the chancre heals, the secondary syphilis stage occurs. Malaise and fatigue, a generalized rash that often includes the palms and soles, wart-like lesions around the genitalia and anus that are flat and moist (condylomata lata), and whitish mucous patches in the mouth are characteristic. This stage also spontaneously resolves and after a period of years, the third stage of syphilis infection, tertiary syphilis, occurs. In this stage, any/every body organ system can be infected, with development of "gummas" - foci of tissue destruction due to hypersensitivity responses to the organism. Gummas can become quite large, and as a result, very destructive. Tertiary syphilis leading to serious complications in the cardiovascular and neurological systems is well recognized.

Syphilis can be transmitted to the fetus at any time during pregnancy. Transmission early in pregnancy can be associated with intrauterine death. Congenital syphilis infection may be asymptomatic or obvious at birth. Its clinical manifestations can include hepatosplenomegaly, dermal erythropoiesis, "pneumonia alba," hepatitis, and long bone changes (periostitis, osteochondritis). Within the first month after birth, additional manifestations can appear: skin fissures and diffuses rashes, mucous discharge from the nose ("snuffles"), jaundice, hemolytic anemia, and mucous patches. If left untreated, longer term effects due to chronic inflammation in the bones, teeth, and central nervous system occur.

Diagnosis

T. pallidum cannot be easily cultured. Therefore, antibody-based screening and diagnosis is the foundation for identification of syphilis. Antibody tests are of two types: specific tests that use actual *T. pallidum* antigens for detection, and reagenic tests - those that use non-*T. pallidum* antigens (which antibodies against *T. pallidum* usually cross-react with) for detection. The former (tests called TPI, FTA-ABS, and MHA-TP) are used to confirm the accuracy of the latter. For general screening, the non-*T.pallidum* tests are used because they are inexpensive. Two tests are widely used: the VDRL (Venereal Disease Research Laboratory) test and the RPR (Rapid Plasma Reagin) test. The VDRL is used to test spinal fluid, and the RPR is used to test serum. To confirm that a positive reagenic test indicates presence of antibody against *T. pallidum*, a specific test is performed once. If it is also positive, it confirms the accuracy of the reagenic test, and the reagenic test is then used to follow response to therapy. Lumbar puncture with VDRL testing of the spinal fluid is done whenever neurosyphilis is considered.

Screening for syphilis should be part of routine prenatal care and should be repeated in high-risk mothers. Infants are considered to be at high risk for congenital syphilis when:

- They are born to a mother with syphilis that was untreated throughout pregnancy.
- There was inadequate response to treatment of the pregnant mother, or she re-acquired new infection.
- They show clinical or radiographic evidence of infection at birth.
- They have a positive cerebrospinal fluid (CSF) VDRL or have abnormal CSF findings with a negative VDRL.
- The infant's RPR titer is more than four-fold higher than the mother's RPR titer.

Treatment

T. pallidum remains sensitive to penicillin, and this drug is still the most dependable treatment for syphilis. The duration of penicillin treatment depends on the stage of disease. Response to treatment is gauged by following changes in serum and spinal fluid levels of antibody using reaginic tests. The presence of one sexually transmitted disease always raises the possibility that others are present. Therefore, individuals with syphilis should also be screened for other STDs (e.g., gonorrhea, HIV, chlamydia, hepatitis B, venereal warts, and HSV). Sexual contacts should also be screened/ treated as appropriate.

Breastfeeding and Syphilis

Because open syphilis lesions are infectious, a mother and/or newborn with open lesions should be separated from one another and from other mothers and infants for 24 hours after treatment with penicillin has been initiated. Although there are no documented cases of transmission of *T. pallidum* from mother to infant via human milk, the propensity of the organism to involve any tissue suggests that human milk transmission is a clear theoretical possibility, and wisdom would dictate that the mother with syphilis should be on treatment at least 24 hours before nursing is allowed. Transmission of syphilis from infant to breast has been documented in an instance where a child with congenital syphilis and oral lesions passed the infection to a wet nurse via the breast (Hamel, 1950).

Summary

The mother and infant with syphilis can breastfeed after they have been on appropriate treatment for syphilis for at least 24 hours.

Reference

Hamel J. Primary chancre of the left breast after multiple suckling of an unrelated syphlitic infant. Dermatol Wochenschr 121:303, 1950.

Toxoplasmosis

Toxoplasma gondii, the causative agent of toxoplasmosis, is a single-celled organism that can cause infection in any human tissue. It is recognized most frequently in three situations: when it causes congenital infection in the fetus, when it infects the brain in the immunocompromised patient, and when toxoplasma retinitis occurs.

T. gondii infection is extremely common, but usually asymptomatic. The definitive host for *T. gondii* is the cat, which usually shows no evidence of infection, but sheds the infective form, the oocyst, in its stool. Contact with cats or cat-contaminated environments (litter boxes, unwashed garden products) is a major source for acquisition, but it can also be acquired by eating under cooked meats that contain *Toxoplasma* cysts. Ingestion is followed by a phase of tissue spread and invasion. In the immunologically competent host, this phase is usually minimally symptomatic (mild fever, transient lymph node enlargement) or asymptomatic, and the illness resolves.

Resolution is associated with development of *Toxoplasma* cysts (another developmental form) in the infected tissues which can lay dormant in the tissues for years. As long as immunocompetency is maintained, occasional transformation of the cysts to tachyzoites (the developmental form with capacity to invade and damage any tissue) is immunologically suppressed by the host and the infection remains dormant. If immunity is lost, the transformation from cyst to tachyzoite results in further tissue invasion and damage in the area where the original *Toxoplasma* cysts were deposited. This is the reason that toxoplasmosis is a significant problem in individuals with immunosuppressive illnesses or treatments.

In many countries, acquisition of toxoplasmosis occurs in early childhood and is never recognized. If acquisition of toxoplasmosis is delayed until childbearing age in women, congenital toxoplasmosis can occur. If a pregnant woman acquires toxoplasmosis, the placenta may be involved during the phase of tissue spread and the organism can be passed to the fetus. The fetus is not immunocompetent, so it cannot control the infection: hence, widespread involvement and injury to fetal tissue occurs. The timing of maternal infection in pregnancy is important with regard to the risk of fetal involvement. In first trimester maternal infection, about 25% of fetuses are infected. For second and third trimester infections, this rate rises to 55% and 65%, respectively. The longer the infection is present, the worse the injury to the fetus. First and second trimester infections can lead to fetal death (Goldenberg & Thompson, 2003), while infections acquired in the third trimester are usually less severe.

Signs and Symptoms

Infected neonates may be asymptomatic at birth and only develop manifestations after some time or may have clinical findings indicative of congenital infection (hepatosplenomegaly, intracranial calcifications, thrombocytopenia). Congenital toxoplasmosis can also produce chorioretinitis, microcephaly, hydrocephalus, seizures, and hepatitis. Sequelae of congenital infection include mental retardation, spasticity, seizures, impaired vision, hearing deficits, and focal muscle weakness.

Treatment

Once an infant with congenital toxoplasmosis is born and begins to develop immunocompetency, it will eventually bring the toxoplasmosis infection under control. However, the damage done *in utero* and ongoing damage after birth while immunocompetency develops usually result in significant deficits.

Treatment of congenital toxoplasmosis usually involves prolonged therapy with sulfadiazine and pyrimethamine: this treatment does not usually stop the infection and its ongoing injury immediately.

Most cases of toxoplasmosis acquired after birth do not require treatment.

Preventing the pregnant woman from acquiring *T. gondii* infection is a much more effective approach than trying to treat congenital toxoplasmosis. Women of child-bearing age should be educated about the risks. Pregnant women should be advised to avoid all contact with cat litter boxes, practice good hand washing after outside activities (e.g., gardening), wash all garden products well, avoid cross-contamination of foods by raw meat, and avoid eating under cooked or raw meats. Prenatal screening for *toxoplasma* antibodies is commonly done, but this is more to help with management because treatment of pregnant women with newly acquired toxoplasmosis has little effect on fetal outcome (Goldenberg & Thompson, 2003; Lopez et al., 2000).

Diagnosis

In the infant suspected to have congenital toxoplasmosis, testing for the presence of IgA and IgM antibody against *T. gondii* is the diagnostic test used. IgM and IgA antibodies do not cross the placenta, so their presence in the infant indicates they are being produced by the infant in response to infection.

Breastfeeding and Toxoplasmosis

A mother and baby with toxoplasmosis can breastfeed.

Summary

Pregnant women should avoid all contact with cat litter boxes; practice good hand washing after outside activities, such as gardening; wash all garden products well before consumption; avoid cross-contamination of foods by raw meat; and avoid consumption of under-cooked or raw meats. Acquisition of infection during pregnancy can have significant effects on the fetus, including fetal death. Mothers with toxoplasmosis can breastfeed, and it is safe for infants with toxoplasmosis to consume human milk.

References

Goldenberg RL, Thompson C. The infectious origins of stillbirth. Am J Obstet Gynecol 189:861-873, 2003.

Lopez A, Dietz VJ, Wilson M, Navin TR, Jones JL. Preventing congenital toxoplasmosis. MMWR 49(RR-2):59-68, 2000.

Tracheoesophageal Fistula (TE Fistula)

Esophageal atresia, with or without tracheoesophageal fistula, occurs in 1:2000 to 1:5000 births. The most common form, occurring in about 85% of cases, is a proximal esophageal pouch and a fistula connecting the trachea to the distal esophagus.

Signs and Symptoms

In a newborn infant, copious oral secretions with respiratory distress and possible aspiration is the symptom constellation that suggests TE fistula. Failure to pass a nasogastric tube is suggestive, and if an x-ray examination of the infant reveals the feeding tube coiled in the esophageal pouch, this confirms the diagnosis. Maternal polyhydramnios during pregnancy is present in about 50% of cases.

Treatment

The treatment of TE fistula is surgical and is focused on removal of the fistulous connection between the esophagus and trachea and reestablishment of esophageal continuity. If possible, primary re-anastamosis of the esophagus is most desirable, but sometimes other approaches are needed, such as chronic elongation of the esophagus before re-anastamosis or use of the stomach, colon, or other tissues to replace or reconstruct the missing esophageal segment. If the infant is otherwise healthy, surgical repair may be attempted immediately following diagnosis. However, if complications from failed feeding or aspiration pneumonia occur, they may need to be resolved before repair is attempted. During recovery from surgery, it is common to maintain the infant in a head-elevated position.

Breastfeeding and TE Fistula

There is nothing about TE fistula per se that is a contraindication to breastfeeding or human milk feeding specifically. Once a TE fistula is recognized, all oral feeding is stopped and feeding is supplied via gastric tube to prevent aspiration pneumonia or other complications. Human milk can certainly provide the calories needed for healing following surgical repair, but usually feeding after esophageal anastamosis surgery continues via gastric tube to avoid contamination of the esophageal wound until it is healed. Thus, feeding at the breast may not be appropriate for some time after surgery. During this time, the mother should be encouraged to pump both to maintain her milk supply and to provide her milk to her infant.

Summary

The infant with a TE fistula may not be allowed to take any nourishment by mouth until the defect is repaired. In this case, feeding of mother's milk via gastric tube is appropriate. The mother should be encouraged to maintain her milk supply by pumping and to use this milk for feeding her infant. Once the child recovers from corrective surgery, breastfeeding can be initiated.

Reference

Houben CH, Curry JI. Current status of prenatal diagnosis, operative management and outcome of esophageal atresia/trachco-csophagcal fistula. Prenat Diagn Feb 27, 2008.

Trichomoniasis

Trichomonas vaginalis is a protozoal parasite that can cause an infection in the adult female genital tract called trichomoniasis. It is a sexually transmitted disease that presents as vaginitis in most women and is asymptomatic in most males. The presence of trichomoniasis in a woman should trigger testing of her and her sexual contacts for other sexually transmitted diseases.

Signs and Symptoms

Trichomonal vaginitis results in foul smelling, frothy, yellowish vaginal discharge, itching and/or dysuria. Vulvovaginal erythema may accompany the discharge. Diagnosis is made by microscopic examination of the vaginal discharge which reveals pear-shaped, motile trichomonads in the wet mount. Culture and antibody testing are infrequently used. Identification of trichomonads on urinanalysis or in Pap smears also occurs.

Treatment

Metronidazole (Flagyl) treatment as a single 2-gram dose for adults or adolescents has about 95% effectiveness as treatment for trichomoniasis. Sexual partners should be treated at the same time, even if they are asymptomatic.

Breastfeeding and Trichomoniasis Medications

Metronidazole is an antibiotic used widely for treatment of anaerobic infections and is also used for treatment of pediatric giardiasis. Metronidazole is not FDA approved for use in children less than two years of age. Currently, its use in breastfeeding mothers is controversial. This is why the Redbook 2006 published by the American Academy of Pediatrics states that metronidazole is an *in vitro* mutagen and, although its effects on the breastfeeding infant are unknown, they may be of concern. Therefore, it may be appropriate to discontinue breastfeeding for 12 to 24 hours to allow excretion when single dose therapy is given to the mother (American Academy of Pediatrics, 2006). While toxicity of metronidazole for human infants has never been definitively demonstrated, neither has its complete safety. Therefore, it is reasonable to avoid exposing the nursing infant to it when possible. To this end, a mother treated with metronidazole, 2 grams as one dose for trichomoniasis, should consider pumping and discarding her milk over the 24 hours following the dose.

Breastfeeding and Trichomoniasis

The mother with trichomoniasis can breastfeed. The mother treated with metronidazole for this condition should not feed her infant her milk for approximately 24 hours following medication dosing.

Summary

The mother with trichomoniasis can breastfeed. The mother treated with metronidazole for this condition should not feed her infant her milk for approximately 24 hours following medication dosing.

Reference

American Academy of Pediatrics. Antimicrobial Agents in Human Milk. In: Pickering LK, Baker CJ, Long SS, McMillan JA, eds. Redbook: 2006 Report of the Committee on Infectious Diseases. 27th edition. Elk Grove Village, IL: American Academy of Pediatrics, 2006: pp 128-130.

Tuberculosis

Tuberculosis is the disease that results from infection with *Mycobacterium tuberculosis*. It is a disease with a long history of causing death and misery for humans, and world wide, it remains a significant cause of infectious disease morbidity and mortality. Most frequently, *M. tuberculosis* is transmitted from human to human by respiratory droplets generated when an individual with pulmonary infection participates in any activity that generates a fine particulate aerosol: coughing, sneezing, singing, even playing brass instruments. The droplets are inhaled by others and deposited in the alveoli of the lung, where the tuberculosis organisms multiply. In the lung, the multiplying organisms are either handled by the host's defenses or go on to cause disease. Active clinical disease occurs in only about 5% of normal individuals who inhale *M. tuberculosis* organisms, but the other 95% of people carry the organism for life and have the potential to develop active disease later in life if they are not recognized and treated.

An individual with tuberculosis infection can be either asymptomatic or symptomatic with tuberculosis disease. Tuberculosis infection is diagnosed by a positive tuberculin skin test reaction. An individual with tuberculosis disease, in addition to usually having a positive skin test, has additional findings that indicate disease: an abnormal chest x-ray, a sputum that shows the organisms by stain or culture, or some other evidence of organ involvement.

Mothers with active pulmonary tuberculosis at the time of delivery are a very significant threat to their infants because young infants are prone to development of disease when they acquire infection. Active, untreated pulmonary tuberculosis in a new mother is considered an indication to separate the infant from the mother until the mother and infant have been started on antituberculous therapy, the mother agrees to wear a mask, and the mother understands and agrees to adhere to proper infection control measures. In the case of suspected multi-drug resistant *M. tuberculosis* in the mother, the infant should be separated from the mother until an expert in tuberculosis disease treatment has been consulted (American Academy of Pediatrics, 2006).

Signs and Symptoms

Tuberculosis is one of the conditions referred to as a "great pretender," meaning that its clinical manifestations can mimic any other disease.

However, most transmission of tuberculosis results from contact with an individual with active lung disease, and this is usually manifested by cough, sputum production, fever, weight loss, and malaise. Chest x-ray of such an individual usually shows pulmonary infiltrate, with or without lymphadenopathy, and sometime pleural effusion. Spread of infection to organs outside the lungs is always a consideration, and any organ system can be infected by *M. tuberculosis*.

Treatment

Treatment of tuberculosis is determined by the severity of the infection and the ability of the drugs used to treat the infection. Infection without any clinical manifestations (e.g., only a positive skin test) is usually treated with one drug. Pulmonary disease with cavity formation is treated initially with three drugs and then tapered to two drugs. Cavitary pulmonary disease and tuberculous meningitis are often treated with four drugs and then tapered to three. The presence or risk of antibiotic resistance in the strain causing infection and/or disease further modifies the treatment regimen, usually causing addition of more treatment drugs. Because treatment of tuberculosis can be confusing and complex, management of the condition is often done by specialists in this condition.

Breastfeeding and Tuberculosis Medications

Most of the medications that the mother takes for treatment of tuberculosis pass into her milk, but the amounts that are transferred to the infant are inadequate for treatment if the infant acquires tuberculosis. Isoniazid, ethambutol, rifampin, and streptomycin are all medications used for treatment of tuberculosis in infants and children, and they are approved for use in breastfeeding women by the American Academy of Pediatrics. Pyrazinamide has not been reviewed, but milk levels are thought to be low.

Breastfeeding and Tuberculosis

A woman with a history of tuberculosis infection (a positive skin test and negative chest x-ray) may breastfeed. A woman with active pulmonary tuberculosis who is untreated should be separated from her infant until she has been on treatment for 14 days. During that period, the mother should pump to maintain her milk supply, and the milk can be used to feed her infant (tuberculosis is usually spread by respiratory droplets, not through breastmilk).

There is no problem with having a skin test for tuberculosis performed during either pregnancy or when breastfeeding, and neither situation modifies the reactivity of the test.

Summary

Active pulmonary tuberculosis without treatment in a breastfeeding mother is a significant threat to her newborn infant and warrants separation of mother and infant. Following initiation of treatment for 14 days, the mother with tuberculosis or a positive skin test can breastfeed. Most of the medications used for treatment of tuberculosis in a mother would also be used for treatment in an infant and, therefore, their transfer in human milk is safe for the infant. However, the amounts transferred in human milk are inadequate for treatment of tuberculosis in the infant.

Reference

American Academy of Pediatrics. Tuberculosis. In: Pickering LK, ed. Red Book: 2006 Report of the Committee on Infectious Diseases. 27th ed. Elk Grove Village, IL: American Academy of Pediatrics, 2006: p 695.

Ulcerative Colitis

Ulcerative colitis is one of the inflammatory bowel diseases, which as its name implies, is restricted to involvement of the colon and rectum. It likely results from a combination of genetic and environmental factors, but its specific cause is unknown. It occurs with an incidence of about 15/100,000, and its prevalence is about equal in males and females. Peaks of disease are seen in the second to third, and fifth to sixth decades of life.

In theory, ulcerative colitis is distinct from Crohn's disease, but practically speaking, about 15% of cases share characteristics. Epidemiologic surveys suggest that the risk of developing inflammatory bowel disease/ ulcerative colitis can be higher (Baron et al., 2005; Jantchou et al., 2005) or lower (Klement et al., 2004) in individuals who were breastfed as infants. The reality is that the effect of breastfeeding on this condition is unclear, but everyone agrees that with its other well-documented benefits, breastfeeding is appropriate in all infants (Jantchou et al., 2005).

Signs and Symptoms

Ulcerative colitis frequently begins at the rectum/anus and spreads proximally. Presenting complaints of bloody/mucousy diarrhea are typical for patients. Longer term manifestations of anemia and hypoalbuminemia can occur, as can more distant manifestations, such as hepatitis, ankylosing spondylitis, sclerosing cholangitis, and pyoderma gangrenosum. In all forms of inflammatory bowel disease in children, growth arrest is common. The grave complication of toxic megacolon occurs in less than 5% of patients with ulcerative colitis.

Diagnosis

No single test is diagnostic for ulcerative colitis. A combination of historical details, physical and radiographic findings, in combination with laboratory findings are usually used to make the diagnosis.

Treatment

Medical management aimed at controlling symptoms and preventing complications is usually the first treatment and may include anti-inflammatory agents, steroid therapy, rest, a modified diet, and oral antibiotic (sulfasalazine) use.

Ulcerative Colitis Medications and Breastfeeding

Ulcerative colitis is usually managed by a specialist because treatment often needs to be modified as the condition waxes and wanes. According to the American Academy of Pediatrics, sulfasalazine should be used with caution in breastfeeding women. In general, its bioavailability is low, and the levels in human milk are also low. It is considered an anti-rheumatic medication that can be continued through pregnancy and lactation (Temprano et al., 2005). Prednisone use by the breastfeeding woman is approved by the American Academy of Pediatrics because the amount that is transferred to the milk is low. However, a major negative effect of chronic steroid use in children is interference with growth, thus the growth of a nursing infant whose mother is being treated with prednisone should be followed carefully.

Breastfeeding and Ulcerative Colitis

As mentioned above, the most recent data are conflicting with regard to the risk of ulcerative colitis developing in individuals who were breastfed as infants. However, if there is a risk, it is outweighed by the other well-documented benefits of human milk feeding. While it has previously been suggested that some women with IBD experience flares in disease activity in the postpartum period, recent data suggest that this is more likely due to discontinuation of treatment rather than an effect of breastfeeding per se (Kane & LeMieux, 2005).

Summary
The mother with ulcerative colitis can breastfeed. If her treatment regimen involves use of sulfasalazine or prednisone, these medications can be continued.

References

Baron S, Tueck D, Leplat C, Merle V, Gower-Rousseau C, Marti R, et al. Environmental risk factors in paediatric inflammatory bowel disease: a population based case control study. Gut 54:357-363, 2005.

Jantchou P, Turck D, Balde M, Gower-Rousseau C. Breastfeeding and risk of inflammatory bowel disease: results of a pediatric, population-based, case-control study. Am J Clin Nutr 82: 485-486, 2005.

Kane S, LeMieux N. The role of breastfeeding in postpartum disease activity in women with inflammatory bowel disease. Am J Gastroenterol 100:102 105, 2005.

Klement E, Cohen RV, Boxman J, Joseph A, Reif S. Breastfeeding and risk of inflammatory bowel disease: a systematic review with meta-analysis. Am J Clin Nutr 80:1342-1352, 2004.

Temprano KK, Bandlamundi R, Moore TL. Antirheumatic drugs in pregnancy and lactation. Semin Arthritis Rheum 35:112-121, 2005.

Upper Respiratory Infections (URIs)

Upper respiratory infections involve the nose and throat and are caused by a large variety of viral infectious agents, including rhinovirus, adenovirus, influenza virus, parainfluenza virus, respiratory syncytial virus, and coronavirus. These infections most commonly occur during the fall, winter, and early spring, and are spread via contact with infected respiratory droplets that are either inhaled or come in contact with other mucosal surfaces (nose, mouth, eyes). Coughing, sneezing, and poor hygiene (lack of hand washing or contact with contaminated surfaces) are usually responsible for person-to-person spread, and spread within families is very common. In small children, acquisition of colds/URIs is common with daycare attendance, tobacco use at home, lower socioeconomic status, and/or crowded living conditions, and these infections predispose to development of ear infections.

Signs and Symptoms

URIs are usually self-limiting diseases, lasting from five to seven days, that usually have their worst symptoms during the first three to five days. Fever is usually low grade (less than 102°F) or may be absent. Nasal congestion, runny nose, sneezing, coughing, watery eyes, scratchy throat, and loss of appetite may also occur. In small infants, the most prominent symptom may be fussiness. Because viral URIs make infection by bacterial agents easier, bronchitis, pneumonia, or sinusitis can develop secondarily. Thus, if URI symptoms in an infant do not improve after five to seven days or if a high fever develops during the course of a URI, this may be a sign of secondary bacterial infection and warrants contacting a physician.

Treatment

Usually, the treatment for URI is symptomatic: rest, get adequate fluid intake, and keep the nasal passages clear (saline nose drops, bulb suction of the nose, humidification of inspired air, elevation of the head when the infant is on their back) are usually adequate to achieve relief. Avoidance of contact with tobacco smoke is wise. A mild analgesic, such as acetaminophen (Tylenol), may give some symptomatic relief, but decongestants and antihistamines should be avoided in small children because their administration may result in paradoxical hyperactivity responses. Aspirin is usually avoided in children less than 18 years old because of its association with development of Reyes syndrome.

Breastfeeding and URIs

Breastfeeding need not be curtailed or modified during URIs in infants or lactating mothers. Existing data indicate that breastfeeding is associated with fewer infectious episodes in infants, including URIs, but if a mother develops a URI, it is prudent for her to avoid coughing on her infant and to practice careful hygiene as far as her hands and respiratory secretions are concerned. Infants with URI may pull off the breast more frequently during feeding because their nasal congestion makes breathing through their noses more difficult. Bulb suction of the nose just before starting to feed may make feeding easier for the infant. Changing to a more upright feeding position may also help because it promotes drainage of secretions from the nose.

Summary
Breastfeeding should continue when a mother or infant develops a URI.

References

Blaymore Bier JA, Oliver T, Ferguson A, Vohr BR. Human milk reduces outpatient upper respiratory symptoms in premature infants during their first year of life. J Perinatol 22:354-359, 2002.

Chantry CJ, Howard CR, Auinger P. Full breastfeeding duration and associated decrease in respiratory tract infection in US children. Pediatrics 117:425-432, 2006.

Quigley MA, Kelly YJ, Sacker A. Breastfeeding and hospitalization for diarrheal and respiratory infection in the United Kingdom Millenium Cohort Study. Pediatrics 119:e837-e842, 2007.

Urinary Tract Infections (UTIs)

Urinary tract infections are usually the result of bacterial migration from the external genitourinary tract into the bladder (cystitis), and in some instances, up into the kidneys (pyelonephritis). Occasionally, they result from blood-borne infection that develops in the kidneys first. Urinary tract infections are much more common in females than males because of the shorter length of the urethra in females. Recurrent cystitis is a fairly common problem in women of child-bearing age. Certain activities/conditions predispose to development of UTIs, including pregnancy, urinary tract manipulation/instrumentation (e.g., cystoscopy, bladder catheterization), and sexual intercourse ("honeymoon cystitis"). Urinary tract infections in infants usually trigger examination of urinary tract structure and function to make sure anatomical abnormalities that predispose to development of infection are not present.

Signs and Symptoms
The most common complaints associated with cystitis are pain on urination, frequent urination, low abdominal pain/discomfort, and fever. If infection

of the kidneys is present, chills, nausea, vomiting, and flank tenderness can occur. In infants, urinary tract infection almost always involves both bladder and kidneys, and non-specific signs, such as fever, fussiness, and loss of appetite, are present. In both adults and children, urinary tract infection can spread to become a systemic infection.

Diagnosis

An examination of the urine (urinalysis) and urine culture are performed to diagnose urinary tract infection. Presence of bacteria, white blood cells, and blood in the urine are suggestive of infection, but depending on the method of urine collection, may only indicate a poorly collected specimen. Urine collected by an improperly performed "clean catch" method is not useful for establishing a diagnosis, explaining why brief bladder catheterization to obtain a urine sample is often used. The numbers of organisms present in the urine are important for correct diagnosis, so methods that allow estimation of the number of bacteria in the urine are used routinely when urine cultures are performed.

Treatment

Cystitis can usually be treated with oral antibiotic therapy, while pyelonephritis usually requires initial intravenous treatment, followed by oral treatment. The antibiotic used in either case is usually directed against enteric (from the intestine) organisms pending identification of the specific organisms isolated by urine culture. In instances where the same organism has been repeatedly cultured from recurrent episodes of UTI, it is common for antibiotic treatment to be administered without urine culture or urinalysis. Repeat urine culture after treatment has started is used to assure the urine has been made sterile by treatment.

Breastfeeding and UTIs

Women or infants with urinary tract infection can breastfeed. There is essentially no risk of transmission of infection from mother-to-infant. Antibiotic therapy in the lactating mother usually results in transfer of small amounts of antibiotic into her milk, which are consumed by the infant. In most instances, this is not considered a problem. If, for some reason, the antibiotic used for treatment of the mother poses a risk to the infant, transient discontinuation of breastfeeding during the period of treatment, with the mother pumping to maintain her milk supply, can be used to prevent exposure of the nursing infant to the mother's treatment medication.

Summary

Urinary tract infections are common in women and do not pose a problem with breastfeeding. Transfer of antibiotics used to treat the mother into breastmilk usually occurs, but the amounts are so small they do not usually need to be considered.

Reference

Kaiser J, McPherson V, Kaufmann L. Which UTI therapies are safe and effective during breastfeeding? J Fam Practice 56:225-228, 2007.

Varicella (Chickenpox)

Varicella is a highly contagious disease that usually occurs in childhood. It is caused by a herpesvirus called Varicella-Zoster virus (VZV). Transmission occurs via contact with infectious respiratory secretions (infectivity is present up to 48 hours before the appearance of the chickenpox rash), or by direct contact with the fluid contained in the vesicles that are the chickenpox rash. In the large majority of children, chickenpox is a benign, self-limiting disease that runs a seven to ten day course and results in life-long immunity. Curiously, secondary cases of chickenpox that occur in family members are often more severe than the index case, presumably because the intensity of exposure to VZV is greater when transmission occurs within a family. More severe disease, including varicella pneumonia, occurs in older adolescents, adults, and immunocompromised individuals who develop chickenpox. Chickenpox results in life-long infection with VZV, although in most normal hosts, no further manifestations occur after the case of chickenpox.

In a small subset of individuals who have had chickenpox, as well as some patients who are immunocompromised after their case of chickenpox, reactivation of the infection occurs, with localized manifestations in the skin that are called zoster (or "shingles"). Zoster usually occurs on one side of the body in the distribution of one or more spinal nerves, and its appearance is a rash that looks very much like localized chickenpox. It can be very painful.

Signs and Symptoms

The incubation period for chickenpox is ten to 14 days, but the large majority of cases develop rash 12 days after exposure. The illness begins non-specifically with low grade fever, malaise, and headache, followed shortly thereafter with development of a few nondescript, small, clear fluid vesicles sitting on an erythematous base - the "dew drop on a rose petal." Over the course of several hours, more lesions appear and mature to look more like the flattened vesicular lesions of chickenpox. Over the course of the first five to seven days, multiple crops of lesions occur and mature, resulting in the presence at any given time of skin lesions at all stages of development. Over time, the clear vesicle fluid becomes cloudy, the lesions appear more pustular and then dry up to form a scab on the skin.

The patient is considered infectious until all skin lesions have scabbed over - usually about seven to nine days. Complications of chickenpox are most commonly bacterial superinfection in the skin or soft tissues caused by *S. aureus* or *S. pyogenes*. Development of superinfection is usually indicated by development of a new high fever five to seven days into the illness, or chickenpox skin lesions that change to become painful, pus-filled, or very red. In adults, varicella pneumonia is a severe complication of chickenpox. Post-infectious complications of chickenpox include transient brain effects (ataxia) or transient post-infectious arthritis.

Treatment

In most instances, treatment of chickenpox is symptomatic: rest, adequate fluid intake, acetaminophen for pain/fever, and anti-pruritus (itching) treatments, such as oral diphenhydramine or oatmeal baths. Aspirin should be avoided in children with chickenpox because of its epidemiologic association with subsequent development of Reye's syndrome. Previously, it was felt that non-steroidal anti-inflammatory agent use in chickenpox could result in more severe disease, but this theory has now been discounted. In severe or life-threatening VZV infection, intravenous treatment with acyclovir can be life-saving and is frequently used in adults with chickenpox because of the disease severity and risk of complications in this group. A related medication, valacyclovir, is available in an effective oral preparation and can be used in the treatment of zoster.

As of 1995, a live, attenuated varicella vaccine is available and has become a standard component of the routine childhood immunization schedule, administered to all children as a single dose between twelve and 18 months of age, and to teenagers who have not received the vaccine, as two doses at least four weeks apart. The varicella vaccine is not approved for administration to children less than 12 months of age or to pregnant women, but can be given to lactating women who are at high risk for development of varicella (i.e., have a recent exposure and did not have chickenpox as a child or were never immunized).

Breastfeeding and Varicella

Women with varicella can breastfeed. Transmission of varicella-zoster virus to the infant is difficult to avoid because the mother has been contagious for up to 48 hours before the appearance of the rash. By definition, such an infant has no passive immunity to infection because they have not received any protective maternal antibody from their mother. Varicella-zoster virus DNA can be detected in breastmilk of women with chickenpox (Yoshida et al., 1992) and shingles (Yoshida et al., 1995) - in this instance, only from the breast on the side with shingles. However, in the case of maternal chickenpox, it is unclear and actually immaterial whether the milk can transmit infection because even before the rash appears, exposure from the mother has already occurred. The infant is likely to develop chickenpox eight to ten days after the rash appears on their mother. In most infants, varicella is a self-limiting illness and is handled well; but in adults, particularly pregnant females, it is often a severe and dangerous illness. Both the breastfeeding mother with varicella and her infant should be followed by a clinician.

Summary

Varicella-Zoster virus is the cause of chickenpox and shingles. Transmission of varicella from a mother to her infant is difficult to avoid due to the intimacy of breastfeeding and the development of contagiousness 48 hours before appearance of the rash. The breastfeeding mother-infant pair with varicella should be followed by a clinician.

References

Yoshida M, Yamagami N, Tezuka T, Hondo R. Case report: detection of varicella-zoster virus DNA in maternal milk. J Med Virol 38:108-110, 1992.

Yoshida M, Tezuka T, Hiruma M. Detection of varicella-zoster virus DNA in maternal breast milk from a mother with herpes zoster. Clin Diagn Virol 4:61-65, 1995.

Glossary

Abscess ....Localized collection of puss.

Ad libitum ....Latin term meaning "at ones pleasure." In medical terms, it refers to giving free access or as much as one desires to use.

Anencephaly ....A neural tube defect caused by failure of the neural tube to close, usually between the 23rd and 26th day of pregnancy, resulting in the absence of a major portion of the brain, skull, and scalp.

Blepharitis ....Inflammation of the eyelids.

Ankylosing ....Caused by or emanating from a fixation of the joint.

Botulinum toxin ....A neurotoxin protein produced by Clostridium botulinum. It is one of the most poisonous naturally occurring substances in the world.

Bradycardia ....A resting heart rate of under 60 beats per minute.

Cervical adenitis...............An inflammation of a lymph node in the neck.

Cervical adenopathy .....Swollen/enlarged lymph nodes in the cervix.

Cervicitis ....An inflammation of the tissues of the cervix

Chalasia ....A condition where the stomach contents flow back up the esophasus. Also called gastroesophageal reflux.

Chancre ....A painless ulceration formed during the primary stage of syphilis.

Chorioretinitis ....An inflammation of the choroid and retina of the eye, also known as choroid retinitis.

Conjunctivitis ....An inflammation of the conjunctiva (outermost layer of the eye and inner surface of the eyelids, also known as pink eye.

Craniotabes ....Abnormal softening or thinning of the skull.

Cystitis ....Inflammation of the urinary bladder.

Cytokine inhibitors ....Substances that inhibit the production of inflammatory cytokines in the body.

Cytotoxic agents ....Substances that are toxic to cells.

Dactylitis ....Sausage-shaped swelling of the fingers and toes.

Dermal erythropoiesis..Abnormal collections of blood forming cells in the skin.

Diabetes mellitus............A syndrome characterized by disordered metabolism and high blood sugar, resulting from either low levels of insulin or from an abnormal resistance to insulin's effects coupled with inadequate levels of insulin secretion.

Dysentery ....Frequent, small-volume, severe diarrhea that shows blood in the feces along with intestinal cramping and painful straining to pass stools.

Dysphagia ....Difficulty swallowing.

Exudative tonsillitis......Infectious inflammation of the tonsils in which the tonsils have a coating of white patches (pus).

Fetid breath ....Bad breath.

Frontal bossing..............Unusually prominent forehead.

Galactose ....Sugar found in breastmilk, dairy products, sugar beets, and other gums and mucilages.

Glossitis ....Inflammation or infection of the tongue. It causes the tongue to swell and change color.

Glossopexy ....A procedure that attaches the tongue to the lower lip and mandible for anterior lingual positioning to resolve upper airway obstruction.

Glossoptosis ....Downward displacement or retraction of the tongue.

Gummas ....Soft, tumor-like growths of tissues, appearing during late-stage syphilis. They usually contain a mass of dead and swollen fiber-like tissue and can occur in any tissue.

Hemolytic anemia.........A condition where there are not enough red blood cells in the blood, caused by premature destruction of red blood cells.

Hepatosplenomegaly...Simultaneous enlargement of both the liver and the spleen.

Herpes simplex virus....A family of viruses that produce life-long infections in humans.

Homcostasis ....The ability of an organism or cell to maintain internal equilibrium by adjusting its physiological processes.

Hydrocephalus...............A condition sometimes known as "water in the brain." It is usually due to blockage of cerebrospinal fluid outflow in the ventricles or in the subarachnoid space over the brain.

Hydrophobia ....Irrational fear of water, to drink or to swim in.

Hyperbilirubinemia......Increased levels of bilirubin in the blood.

Hypernatremia...............Electrolyte imbalance – elevated sodium level in the blood.

Hypertrophy ....Growth and increase in size.

Hypoalbuminemia........Condition where levels of albumin in blood serum are abnormally low.

Intracranial calcification. The hardening of organic tissue within the cranium by a deposit of calcium salts.

Ischemia ....A restriction in blood supply generally due to factors in the blood vessels causing damage or dysfunction of tissue.

Knock-knees ....A condition in which the lower legs are at an outward angle so that when the knees are touching, the ankles are separated.

Mandibular distraction..Surgery of the mandible to relieve airway obstruction.

Mastitis ....Inflammation of the mammary gland or breast.

Mastoiditis ....Inflammation of the mastoid sinus.

Meningomyelocele........A congenital defect characterized by the protrusion of the membranes and cord through a defect in the vertebral column.

Microcephaly ....An abnormally small head of a newborn, a congenitally small brain.

Mucolytics ....Destroying or dissolving mucin, a mucopolysaccharide or glycoprotein that is a chief constituent of mucus.

Osteomyelitis ....Inflammation of bone caused by a pyogenic organism.

Otitis media ....Ear infection.

Palatal abnormalities....Abnormalities of the roof of the mouth.

Palatal petechiae ....Small red or purple spots on the roof of the mouth.

Panhypopituitarism ...... A condition of inadequate or absent production of the anterior pituitary hormones.

Perihepatitis .... Inflammation of the peritoneum and tissues surrounding the liver.

Perineum .... The portion of the body in the pelvis occupied by urogenital passages and the rectum, bounded in front by the pubic arch, in the back by the coccyx, and laterally by part of the hipbone.

Peritonsillar abscess ..... An infection that forms in the tissues of the throat next to one of the tonsils. It is the most common abscess of the head and neck region.

Photophobia .... Abnormal sensitivity and discomfort from light.

Pigeon breast .... A chest deformity marked by a projecting sternum, often occurring as a result of infantile rickets. Also called chicken breast.

Pneumonia alba .... A fatal desquamative pneumonia of the newborn due to congenital syphilis, with fatty degeneration of the lungs.

Pyelonephritis .... Inflammation of the kidney and its pelvis, caused by bacterial infection. Also called nephropyelitis.

Pyloromyotomy .... Longitudinal incision through the anterior wall of the pylorus muscle to the level of the submucosa, performed as a treatment for hypertrophic pyloric stenosis.

Pyoderma gangrenosuma .... Chronic skin disease, usually of the trunk, characterized by large spreading ulcers.

Rachitic rosary .... A row of beadlike prominences at the junction of a rib and its cartilage, often seen in rachitic children. Also called beading of ribs.

Salpingitis .... An infection and inflammation in the fallopian tubes.

Sclera .... The white matter of the eyeball. In the disease osteogenesis imperfecta, the sclera has a bluish color and in hyperbilirubinemia, the sclera is often yellow (jaundiced).

Sclerosing cholangitis .. Hardening of the bile duct due to inflammation.

Secondary adrenal failure ....Occurs when a lack of secretion of corticotrophin-releasing hormone (CRH) from the hypothalamus or of corticotropic hormone (ACTH) from the pituitary leads to hypofunction of the adrenal cortex.

Secondary hypothyroidism ....Condition where the activity of the thyroid gland is decreased, due to failure of the pituitary gland.

Sinusitis ....Inflammation of the paranasal sinuses.

Spina bifida ....A birth defect caused by an incomplete closure of one of more vertebral arches of the spine.

Spondylitis ....Inflammation of a vertebra.

Stomatitis ....Inflammation of the mucous lining of any of the structures in the mouth.

Tracheoesophageal fistula ......A birth defect in which the upper esophagus ends and does not connect with the lower esophagus and stomach. The top end of the lower esophagus connects to the windpipe. This connection is called a tracheoesophageal fistula (TE fistula).

Thrombocytopenia ....The presence of relatively few platelets in blood.

Toxoplasmosis ....A parasitic disease caused by the protozoan, *Toxoplasma gondii*. The parasite infects most warm-blooded animals, but the primary host is the feline (cat) family. The cyst form of the parasite is extremely hardy; however, it is killed by thorough cooking or by freezing. Treatment is very important for recently infected pregnant women to prevent infection of the fetus.

Tracheostomy ....Surgical procedure on the neck to open a direct airway through an incision in the trachea.

Transcutaneous ....By way of or through the skin.

Transglutaminase ....A family of enzymes that catalyze the formation of a covalent bond between a free amine group and the gamma-carboxamid group of protein or peptide-bound glutamine.

Varicella-Zoster virus ... The virus that causes chickenpox and shingles.

Vaso-occlusive .... An obstruction caused by sickle-shaped red blood cells that obstruct capillaries and restrict blood flow to an organ, resulting in restricted blood supply, pain, and organ damage.

Zoster (or "shingles") .. Herpes zoster or shingles is caused by the same virus responsible for chicken pox. It may lie dormant in nerve fibers and become active as a result of aging, stress, suppression of the immune system, and certain medications.

Index

Author Biographies

E. Stephen Buescher, MD, is a Professor of Pediatrics and a member of the Division of Pediatric Basic Sciences. He joined Eastern Virginia Medical School in 1992. Since that time, he has directed a laboratory focused on studies related to inflammation, its cellular and humoral components, and the anti-inflammatory characteristics of human milk.

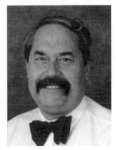

Dr. Buescher practices at Childrens' Hospital of The King's Daughters and is on faculty at Eastern Virginia Medical School. He has a clinical interest in phagocyte functional disorders and is active in medical student teaching. Dr. Buescher's laboratory is currently focused on the characterization and identification of nosocomial infection related organisms and infectious diseases in children and their sequellae.

Susan W. Hatcher, RN, BSN, IBCLC, has been a women's health nurse for nearly twenty years, and an Internationally Board Certified Lactation Consultant since 1992. She has worked in both inpatient and outpatient settings, supporting normal newborns and high risk premature infants. For fifteen years, Susan developed and managed an inpatient and outpatient comprehensive lactation program for a major health

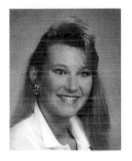

system. She is now in private practice and owner of HealthSource for Women where she focuses on infant oral-motor issues, general feeding difficulties, and maternal problems. Susan also has a passion for professional education and has organized a major lactation conference on the East Coast for the last fifteen years.

ORDERING INFORMATION

HALE PUBLISHING, L.P.
1712 N. FOREST ST.
AMARILLO, TEXAS, USA   79106

8:00 AM TO 5:00 PM CST

ↅ

CALL . 806-376-9900

SALES 800-378-1317

FAX.... 806-376-9901

ↅ

Online Web Orders...

www.ibreastfeeding.com